Alkaline Dessert and Appetizers

A Cookbook for your healthy and sweet Moments

Isaac Vinson

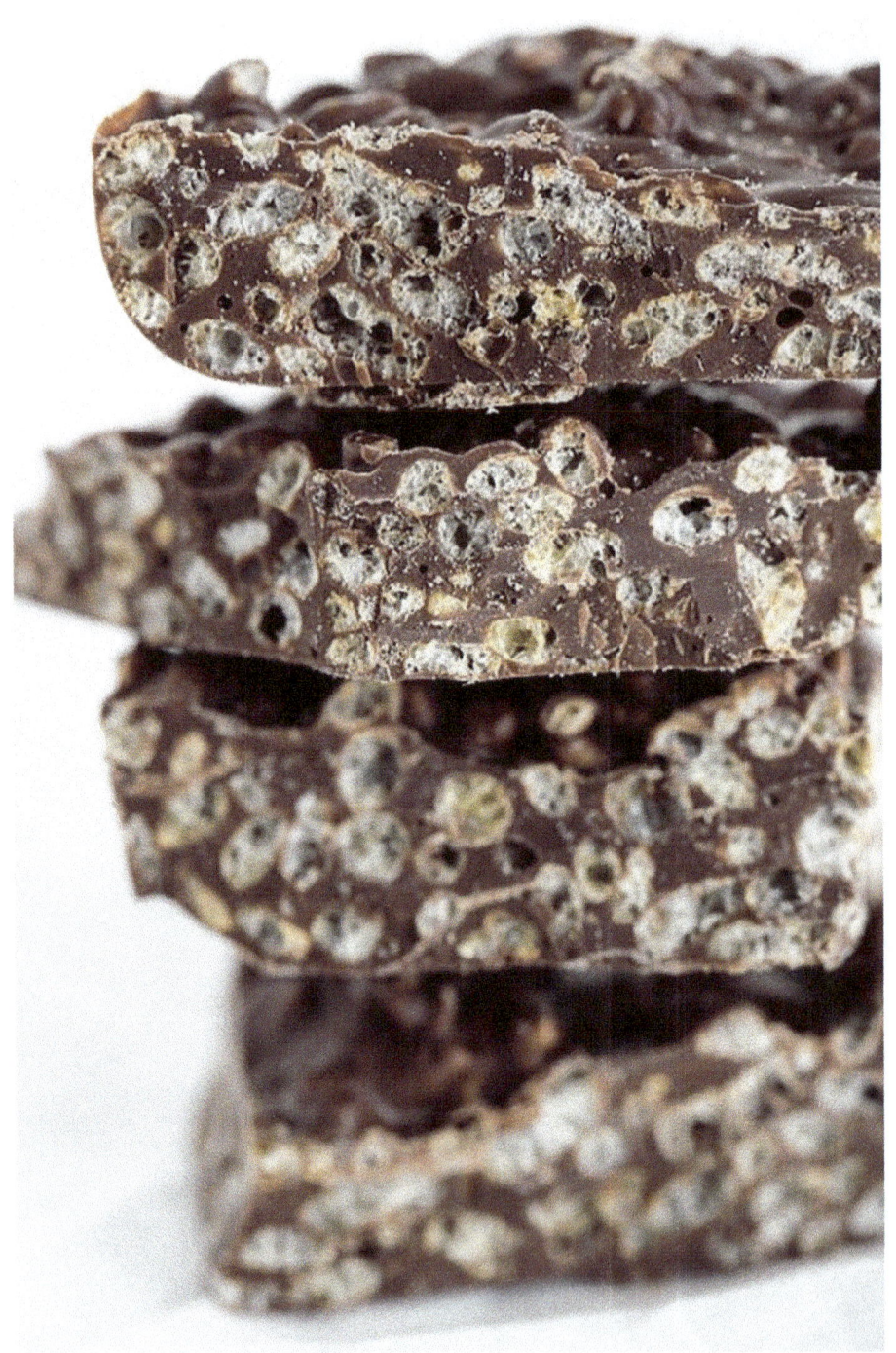

© copyright 2021 – all rights reserved.

the content contained within this book may not be reproduced, duplicated or transmitted without direct written permission from the author or the publisher.

under no circumstances will any blame or legal responsibility be held against the publisher, or author, for any damages, reparation, or monetary loss due to the information contained within this book. either directly or indirectly.

legal notice:

this book is copyright protected. this book is only for personal use. you cannot amend, distribute, sell, use, quote or paraphrase any part, or the content within this book, without the consent of the author or publisher.

disclaimer notice:

please note the information contained within this document is for educational and entertainment purposes only. all effort has been executed to present accurate, up to date, and reliable, complete information. no warranties of any kind are declared or implied. readers acknowledge that the author is not engaging in the rendering of legal, financial, medical or professional advice. the content within this book has been derived from various sources. please consult a licensed professional before attempting any techniques outlined in this book.

by reading this document, the reader agrees that under no circumstances is the author responsible for any losses, direct or indirect, which are incurred as a result of the use of information contained within this document, including, but not limited to, — errors, omissions, or inaccuracies.

Table of Contents

- CHOCOLATE CRUNCH BARS 6
- HOMEMADE PROTEIN BAR 8
- SHORTBREAD COOKIES 11
- COCONUT CHIP COOKIES 13
- PEANUT BUTTER BARS 16
- ZUCCHINI BREAD PANCAKES 18
- BERRY SORBET 21
- QUINOA PORRIDGE 23
- APPLE QUINOA 25
- KAMUT PORRIDGE 28
- HOT KAMUT WITH PEACHES, WALNUTS, AND COCONUT 30
- OVERNIGHT "OATS" 32
- BRAZIL NUT CHEESE 34
- BAKED STUFFED PEARS 36
- BUTTERNUT SQUASH PIE 39
- COCONUT CHIA CREAM POT 41
- CHOCOLATE AVOCADO MOUSSE 44
- CHIA VANILLA COCONUT PUDDING 45
- SWEET TAHINI DIP WITH GINGER CINNAMON FRUIT 48
- COCONUT BUTTER AND CHOPPED BERRIES WITH MINT 50
- ALKALINE RAW PUMPKIN PIE 51
- STRAWBERRY SORBET 54
- BLUEBERRY CUPCAKES 56
- BANANA STRAWBERRY ICE CREAM 58
- HOMEMADE WHIPPED CREAM 60
- "CHOCOLATE" PUDDING 61
- BANANA NUT MUFFINS 63
- BLACKBERRY JAM 65
- BLACKBERRY BARS 68
- DETOX BERRY SMOOTHIE 70
- TABBOULEH- ARABIAN SALAD 72

Aromatic Toasted Pumpkin Seeds 75
Bacon-Wrapped Shrimps 77
Cheesy Broccoli Bites 78
Easy Caprese Skewers 81
Grilled Tofu With Sesame Seeds 82
Kale Chips 84
Simple Deviled Eggs 87
Sautéed Collard Greens And Cabbage 89
Roasted Delicata Squash With Thyme 92
Roasted Asparagus And Red Peppers 94
Tarragon Spring Peas 96
Butter-Orange Yams 98
Roasted Tomato Brussels Sprouts 101
Simple Sautéed Greens 103
Garlicky Mushrooms 104

Chocolate Crunch Bars

Preparation Time: 5 minutes
Cooking Time: 5 minutes
Servings: 4

Ingredients :
- 1 1/2 cups sugar-free chocolate chips

- 1 cup almond butter

- Stevia to taste

- 1/4 cup coconut oil

- 3 cups pecans , chopped

Directions:
1. Layer an 8-inch baking pan with parchment paper.

2. Mix chocolate chips with butter, coconut oil, and sweetener in a bowl.

3. Melt it by heating in a microwave for 2 to 3 minutes until well mixed.

4. Stir in nuts and seeds. Mix gently.

5. Pour this batter carefully into the baking pan and spread evenly.

6. Refrigerate for 20 minutes.

7. Slice and serve.

Nutrition:
Calories 316

Total Fat 30.9 g

Saturated Fat 8.1 g

Cholesterol 0 mg

Total Carbs 8.3 g

Sugar 1.8 g

Fiber 3.8 g

Sodium 8 mg

Protein 6.4 g

Homemade Protein Bar

Preparation Time: 5 minutes
Cooking Time: 10 minutes
Servings: 4

Ingredients :
- 1 cup nut butter

- 4 tablespoons coconut oil

- 2 scoops vanilla protein

- Stevia, to taste

- ½ teaspoon sea salt

- Optional Ingredients

- 1 teaspoon cinnamon

Directions:
1. Mix coconut oil with butter, protein, stevia, and salt in a dish.

2. Stir in cinnamon and chocolate chip.

3. Press the mixture firmly and freeze until firm.

4. Cut the crust into small bars.

5. Serve and enjoy.

Nutrition:
Calories 179

Total Fat 15.7 g

Saturated Fat 8 g

Cholesterol 0 mg

Total Carbs 4.8 g

Sugar 3.6 g

Fiber 0.8 g

Sodium 43 mg

Protein 5.6 g

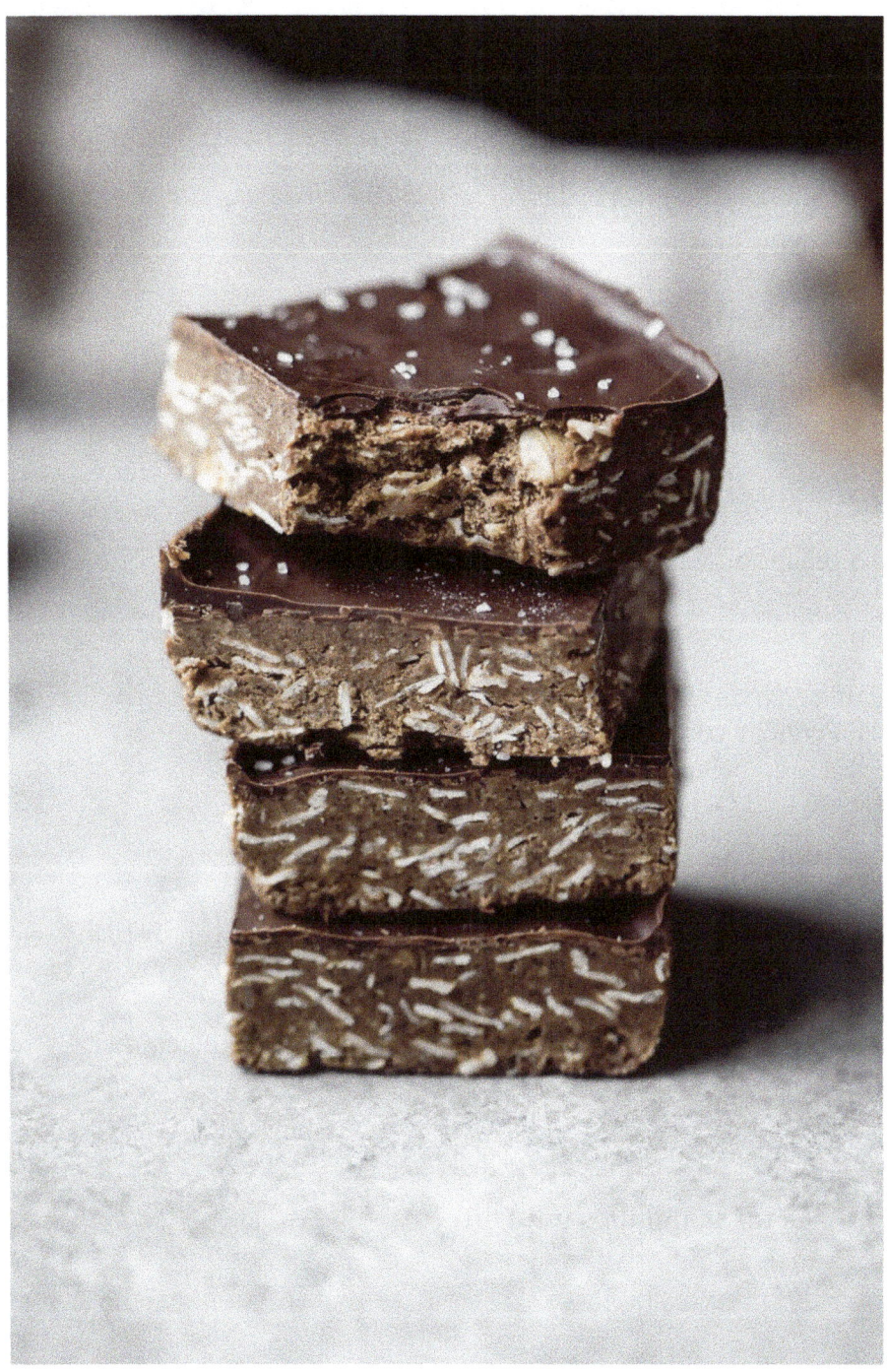

Shortbread Cookies

Preparation Time: 10 minutes
Cooking Time: 70 minutes
Servings: 6

Ingredients :
- 2 1/2 cups almond flour

- 6 tablespoons nut butter

- 1/2 cup erythritol

- 1 teaspoon vanilla essence

Directions:
1. Preheat your oven to 350 degrees F.

2. Layer a cookie sheet with parchment paper.

3. Beat butter with erythritol until fluffy.

4. Stir in vanilla essence and almond flour. Mix well until becomes crumbly.

5. Spoon out a tablespoon of cookie dough onto the cookie sheet.

6. Add more dough to make as many cookies.

7. Bake for 15 minutes until brown.

8. Serve.

Nutrition:
Calories 288

Total Fat 25.3 g

Saturated Fat 6.7 g

Cholesterol 23 mg

Total Carbs 9.6 g

Sugar 0.1 g

Fiber 3.8 g

Sodium 74 mg

Potassium 3 mg

Protein 7.6 g

Coconut Chip Cookies

Preparation Time: 10 minutes
Cooking Time: 15 minutes
Servings: 4

Ingredients :
- 1 cup almond flour

- ½ cup cacao nibs

- ½ cup coconut flakes, unsweetened

- 1/3 cup erythritol

- ½ cup almond butter

- ¼ cup nut butter, melted

- ¼ cup almond milk

- Stevia, to taste

- ¼ teaspoon sea salt

Directions:
1. Preheat your oven to 350 degrees F.

2. Layer a cookie sheet with parchment paper.

3. Add and then combine all the dry Ingredients in a glass bowl.

4. Whisk in butter, almond milk, vanilla essence, stevia, and almond butter.

5. Beat well then stir in dry mixture. Mix well.

6. Spoon out a tablespoon of cookie dough on the cookie sheet.

7. Add more dough to make as many as 16 cookies.

8. Flatten each cookie using your fingers.

9. Bake for 25 minutes until golden brown.

10. Let them sit for 15 minutes.

11. Serve.

Nutrition:
Calories 192

Total Fat 17.44 g

Saturated Fat 11.5 g

Cholesterol 125 mg

Total Carbs 2.2 g

Sugar 1.4 g

Fiber 2.1 g

Sodium 135 mg

Protein 4.7 g

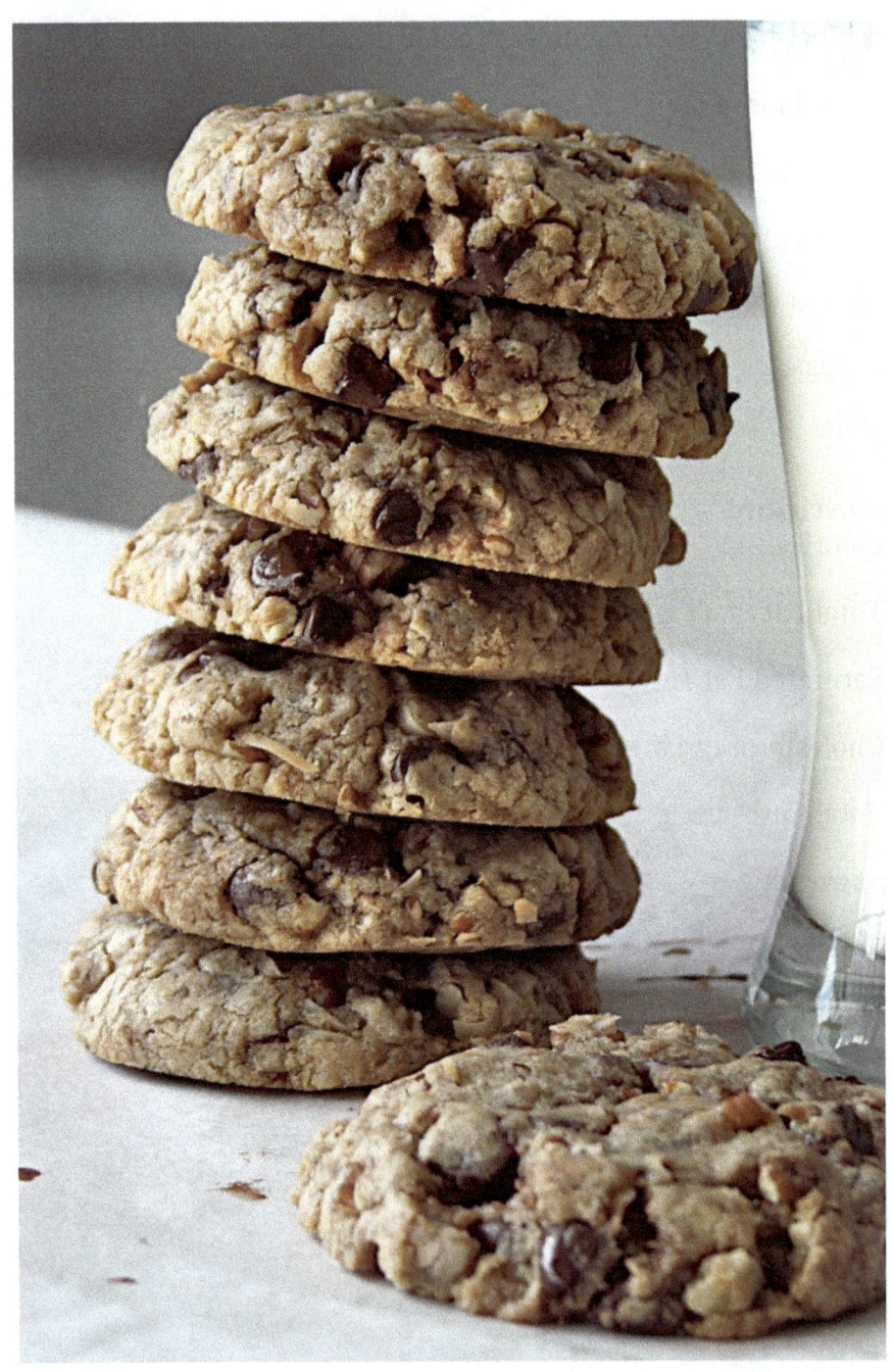

Peanut Butter Bars

Preparation Time: 10 minutes
Cooking Time: 10 minutes
Servings: 6

Ingredients :
- 3/4 cup almond flour

- 2 oz. almond butter

- 1/4 cup Swerve

- 1/2 cup peanut butter

- 1/2 teaspoon vanilla

Directions:
1. Combine all the Ingredients for bars.

2. Transfer this mixture to 6-inch small pan. Press it firmly.

3. Refrigerate for 30 minutes.

4. Slice and serve.

Nutrition:
Calories 214

Total Fat 19 g

Saturated Fat 5.8 g

Cholesterol 15 mg

Total Carbs 6.5 g

Sugar 1.9 g

Fiber 2.1 g

Sodium 123 mg

Protein 6.5 g

Zucchini Bread Pancakes

Preparation Time: 15 minutes
Cooking Time: 35 minutes
Servings: 3

Ingredients :
• Grapeseed oil, 1 tbsp.

• Chopped walnuts, .5 c

• Walnut milk, 2 c

• Shredded zucchini, 1 c

• Mashed burro banana, .25 c

• Date sugar, 2 tbsp.

• Kamut flour or spelt, 2 c

Directions:
1. Place the date sugar and flour into a bowl. Whisk together.

2. Add in the mashed banana and walnut milk. Stir until combined. Remember to scrape the bowl to get all the dry mixture. Add in walnuts and zucchini. Stir well until combined.

3. Place the grapeseed oil onto a griddle and warm.

4. Pour .25 cup batter on the hot griddle. Leave it along until bubbles begin forming on to surface. Carefully turn over the pancake and cook another four minutes until cooked through.

5. Place the pancakes onto a serving plate and enjoy with some agave syrup.

Nutrition:
Calories: 246

Carbohydrates: 49.2 g

Fiber: 4.6 g

Protein: 7.8 g

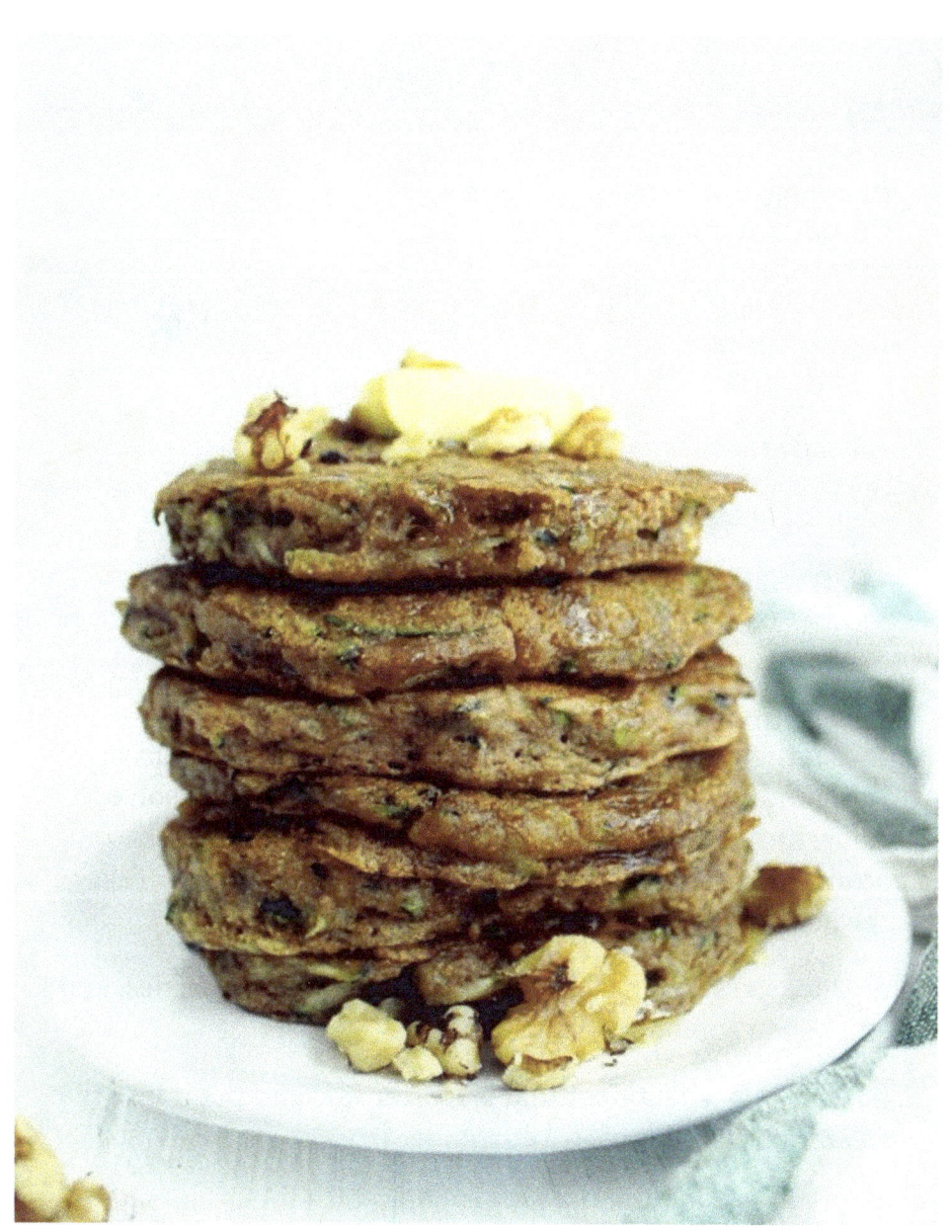

Berry Sorbet

Preparation Time: 10 minutes
Cooking Time: 20 minutes
Servings: 6

Ingredients :
- Water, 2 c

- Blend strawberries, 2 c

- Spelt Flour, 1.5 tsp.

- Date sugar, .5 c

Directions:
1. Add the water into a large pot and let the water begin to warm. Add the flour and date sugar and stir until dissolved. Allow this mixture to start boiling and continue to cook for around ten minutes. It should have started to thicken. Take off the heat and set to the side to cool.

2. Once the syrup has cooled off, add in the strawberries, and stir well to combine.

3. Pour into a container that is freezer safe and put it into the freezer until frozen.

4. Take sorbet out of the freezer, cut into chunks, and put it either into a blender or a food processor. Hit the pulse button until the mixture is creamy.

5. Pour this into the same freezer-safe container and put it back into the freezer for four minutes.

Nutrition:
Calories: 99

Carbohydrates: 8 g

Quinoa Porridge

Preparation Time: 5 minutes
Cooking Time: 15 minutes
Servings: 04

Ingredients :
• Zest of one lime

• Coconut milk, .5 c

• Cloves, .5 tsp.

• Ground ginger, 1.5 tsp.

• Spring water, 2 c

• Quinoa, 1 c

• Grated apple, 1

Directions:
1. Cook the quinoa. Follow the instructions on the package. When the quinoa has been cooked, drain well. Place it back into the pot and stir in spices.

2. Add coconut milk and stir well to combine.

3. Grate the apple now and stir well.

4. Divide equally into bowls and add the lime zest on top. Sprinkle with nuts and seeds of choice.

Nutrition:
Calories: 180

Fat: 3 g

Carbohydrates: 40 g

Protein: 10 g

Apple Quinoa

Preparation Time: 15 minutes
Cooking Time: 30 minutes
Servings: 04

Ingredients :
• Coconut oil, 1 tbsp.

• Ginger

• Key lime .5

• Apple, 1

• Quinoa, .5 c

• Optional toppings

• Seeds

• Nuts

• Berries

Directions:
1. Fix the quinoa according to the instructions on the package. When you are getting close to the end of the Cooking time, grate in the apple and cook for 30 seconds.

2. Zest the lime into the quinoa and squeeze the juice in. Stir in the coconut oil.

3. Divide evenly into bowls and sprinkle with some ginger.

4. You can add in some berries, nuts, and seeds right before you eat.

Nutrition:
Calories: 146

Fiber: 2.3 g

Fat: 8.3 g

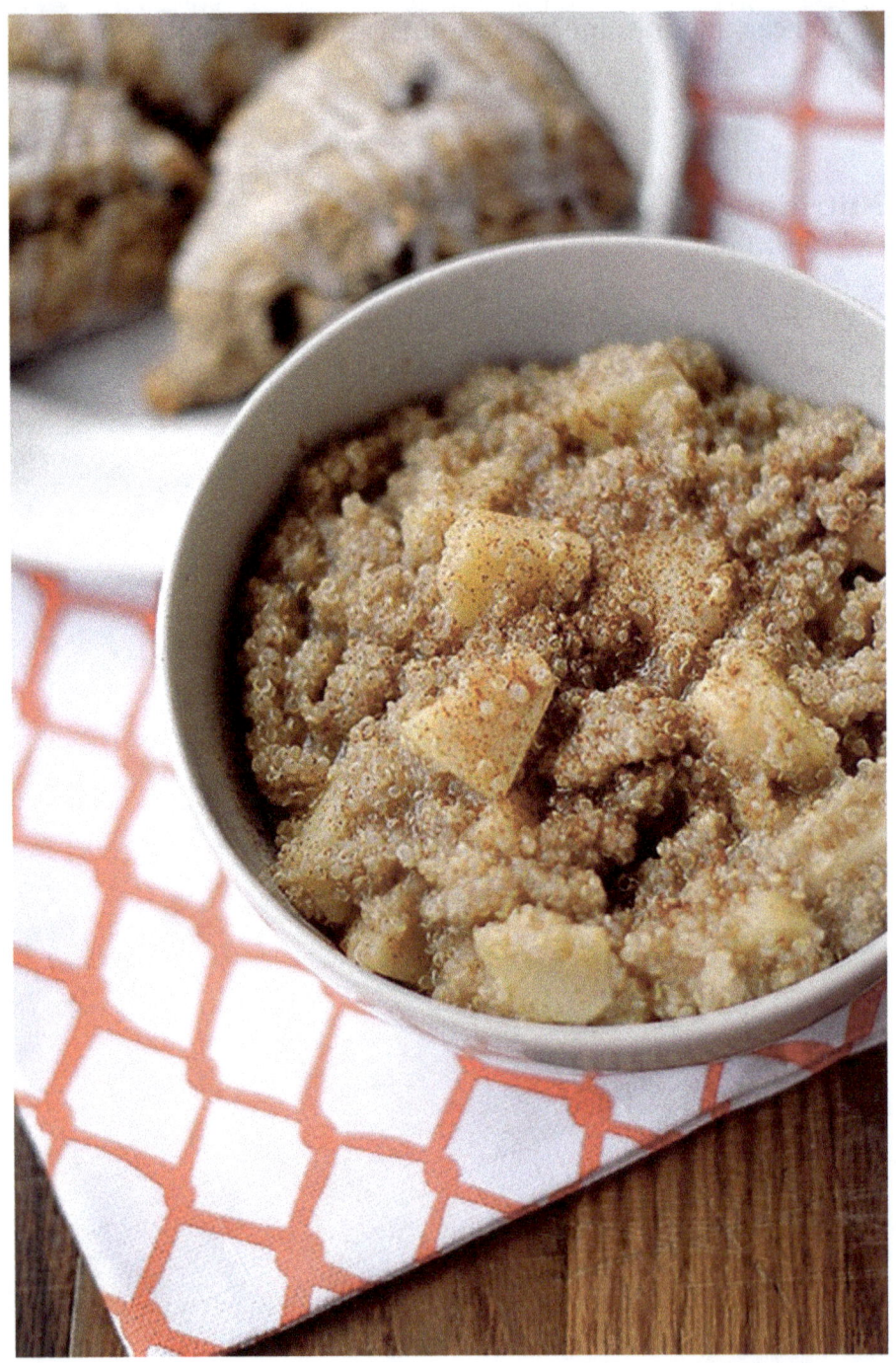

Kamut Porridge

Preparation Time: 10 minutes
Cooking Time: 25 minutes
Servings: 04

Ingredients :
• Agave syrup, 4 tbsp.

• Coconut oil, 1 tbsp.

• Sea salt, .5 tsp.

• Coconut milk, 3.75 c

• Kamut berries, 1 c

• Optional toppings

• Berries

• Coconut chips

• Ground nutmeg

• Ground cloves

Directions:
1. You need to "crack" the Kamut berries. You can try this by placing the berries into a food processor and pulsing until you have **1.** 25 cups of Kamut.

2. Place the cracked Kamut in a pot with salt and coconut milk. Give it a good stir in order to combine everything. Allow this mixture to come to a full rolling boil and then turn the heat down until the mixture is simmering. Stir every now and then until the Kamut has thickened to your likeness. This normally takes about ten minutes.

3. Take off heat, stir in agave syrup and coconut oil.

4. Garnish with toppings of choice and enjoy.

Nutrition:
Calories: 114

Protein: 5 g

Carbohydrates: 24g

Fiber: 4 g

Hot Kamut With Peaches, Walnuts, And Coconut

Preparation Time: 10 minutes
Cooking Time: 35 minutes
Servings: 04

Ingredients :
- Toasted coconut, 4 tbsp.

- Toasted and chopped walnuts, .5 c

- Chopped dried peaches, 8

- Coconut milk, 3 c

- Kamut cereal, 1 c

Directions:
1. Mix the coconut milk into a saucepan and allow it to warm up. When it begins simmering, add in the Kamut. Let this cook about 15 minutes, while stirring every now and then.

2. When done, divide evenly into bowls and top with the toasted coconut, walnuts, and peaches.

3. You could even go one more and add some fresh berries.

Nutrition:
Calories: 156

Protein: 5.8 g

Carbohydrates: 25 g

Fiber: 6 g

Overnight "Oats"

Preparation Time: 5 minutes
Cooking Time: 0 minutes
Servings: 04

Ingredients :
• Berry of choice, .5 c

• Walnut butter, .5 tbsp.

• Burro banana, .5

• Ginger, .5 tsp.

• Coconut milk, .5 c

• Hemp seeds, .5 c

Directions:
1. Put the hemp seeds, salt, and coconut milk into a glass jar. Mix well.

2. Place the lid on the jar then put in the refrigerator to sit overnight.

3. The next morning, add the ginger, berries, and banana. Stir well and enjoy.

Nutrition:
Calories: 139

Fat: 4.1 g

Protein: 9 g

Sugar: 7 g

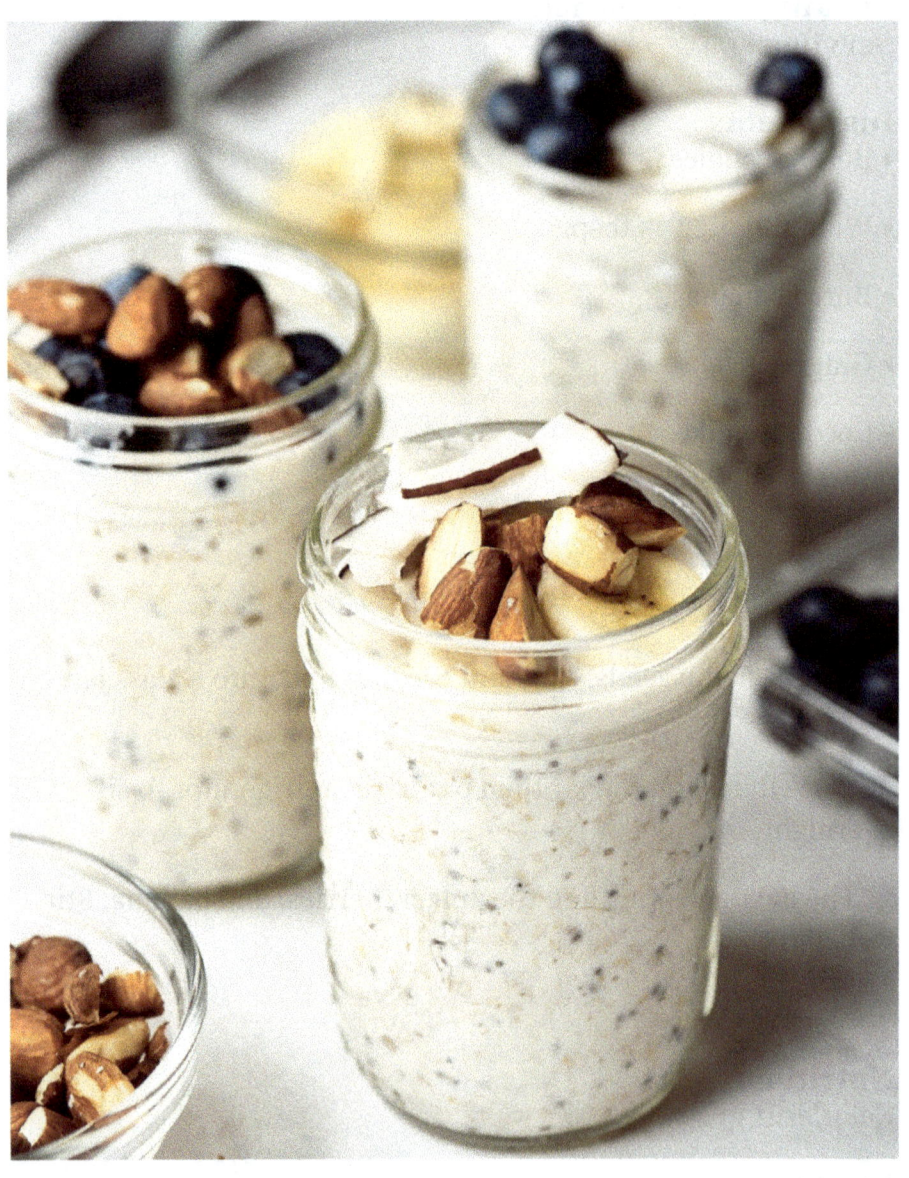

Brazil Nut Cheese

Preparation Time: 20 minutes
Cooking Time: 0 minutes
Servings: 04

Ingredients :
• Grapeseed oil, 2 tsp.

• Water, 1.5 c

• Hemp milk, 1.5 c

• Cayenne, .5 tsp.

• Onion powder, 1 tsp.

• Juice of .5 lime

• Sea salt, 2 tsp.

• Brazil nuts, 1 lb.

• Onion powder, 1 tsp.

Directions:
1. You will need to start process by soaking the Brazil nuts in some water. You just put the nuts into a bowl and make sure the water covers them. Soak no less than 20 minutes or overnight. Overnight would be best.

2. Now you need to put everything except water into a food processor or blender.

3. Add just .5 cups water and blend for two minutes

4. Continue adding .5 cup water and blending until you have the consistency you want.

5. Scrape into an airtight container and enjoy.

Nutrition:
Calories: 187

Protein: 4.1 g

Fat: 19 g

Carbs: 3.3 g

Fiber: 2.1 g

Baked Stuffed Pears

Preparation Time: 15 minutes
Cooking Time: 35 minutes
Servings: 04

Ingredients :
- Agave syrup, 4 tbsp.

- Cloves, .25 tsp.

- Chopped walnuts, 4 tbsp.

- Currants, 1 c

- Pears, 4

Directions:
1. Make sure your oven has been warmed to 375

2. Slice the pears in two lengthwise and remove the core. To get the pear to lay flat, you can slice a small piece off the back side.

3. Place the agave syrup, currants, walnuts, and cloves in a small bowl and mix well. Set this to the side to be used later.

4. Put the pears on a cookie sheet that has parchment paper on it. Make sure the cored sides are facing up. Sprinkle each pear half with about .5 tablespoon of the chopped walnut mixture.

5. Place into the oven and cook for 25 to 30 minutes. Pears should be tender.

Nutrition:
Calories: 103.9

Fiber: 3.1 g

Carbohydrates: 22 g

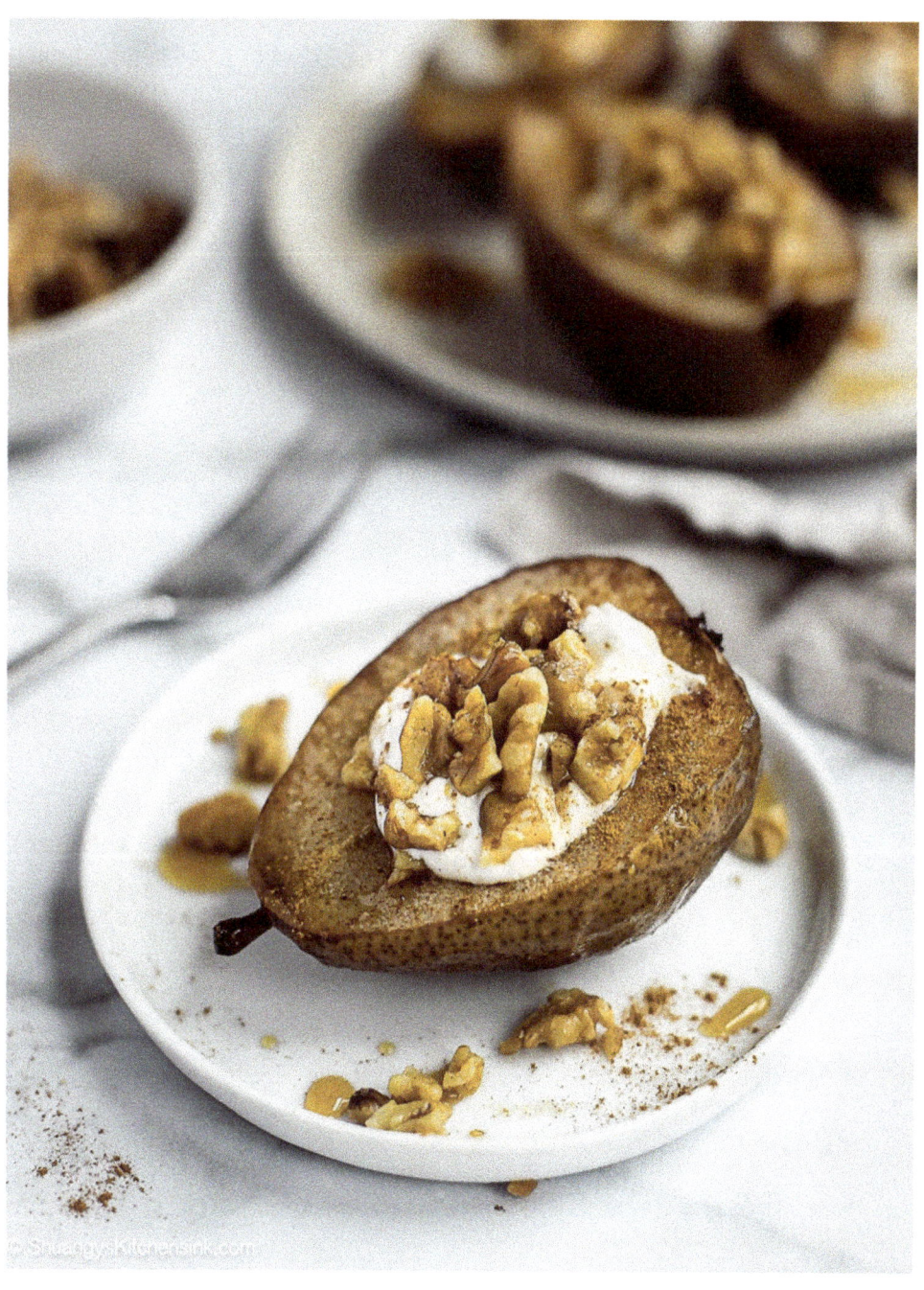

Butternut Squash Pie

Preparation Time: 25 minutes
Cooking Time: 35 minutes
Servings: 04

Ingredients :
• For the Crust

• Cold water

• Agave, splash

• Sea salt, pinch

• Grapeseed oil, .5 c

• Coconut flour, .5 c

• Spelt Flour, 1 c

• For the Filling

• Butternut squash, peeled, chopped

• Water

• Allspice, to taste

• Agave syrup, to taste

• Hemp milk, 1 c

• Sea moss, 4 tbsp.

Directions:
1. You will need to warm your oven to 350.

2. For the Crust

3. Place the grapeseed oil and water into the refrigerator to get it cold. This will take about 10 minutes.

4. Place all Ingredients into a large bowl. Now you need to add in the cold water a little bit in small amounts until a dough forms. Place this onto a surface that has been sprinkled with some coconut flour. Knead for a few minutes and roll the dough as thin as you can get it. Carefully, pick it up and place it inside a pie plate.

5. Place the butternut squash into a Dutch oven and pour in enough water to cover. Bring this to a full rolling boil. Let this cook until the squash has become soft.

6. Completely drain and place into bowl. Using a potato masher, mash the squash. Add in some allspice and agave to taste. Add in the sea moss and hemp milk. Using a hand mixer, blend well. Pour into the pie crust.

7. Place into an oven and bake for about 30 minutes.

Nutrition:
Calories: 245

Carbohydrates: 50 g

Fat: 10 g

Coconut Chia Cream Pot

Preparation Time: 5 minutes
Cooking Time: 5 minutes
Servings: 04

Ingredients :
• Date, one (1)

• Coconut milk (organic), one (1) cup

• Coconut yogurt, one (1) cup

• Vanilla extract, ½ teaspoon

• Chia seeds, ¼ cup

• Sesame seeds, one (1) teaspoon

• Flaxseed (ground), one (1) tablespoon or flax meal, one (1) tablespoon

• Toppings:

• Fig, one (1)

• Blueberries, one(1) handful

• Mixed nuts (brazil nuts, almonds, pistachios, macadamia, etc.)

• Cinnamon (ground), one teaspoon

Directions:
1. First, blend the date with coconut milk (the idea is to sweeten the coconut milk).

2. Get a mixing bowl and add the coconut milk with the vanilla, sesame seeds, chia seeds, and flax meal.

3. Refrigerate for between twenty to thirty minutes or wait till the chia expands.

4. To serve, pour a layer of coconut yogurt in a small glass, then add the chia mix, followed by pouring another layer of the coconut yogurt.

5. It's alkaline, creamy and delicious.

Nutrition:
Calories: 310

Carbohydrates: 39 g

Protein: 4 g

Fiber: 8.1 g

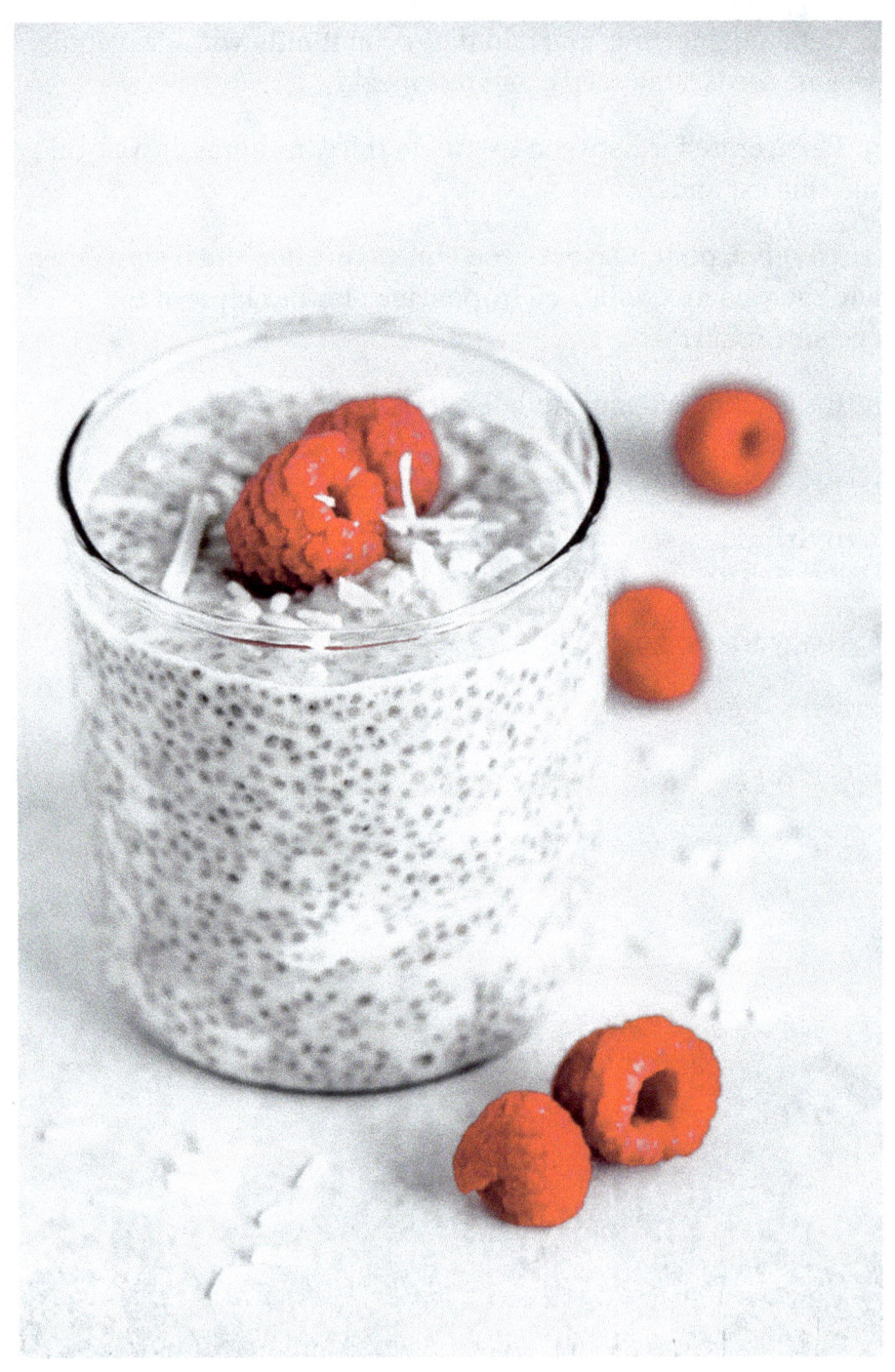

Chocolate Avocado Mousse

Preparation Time: 10 minutes
Cooking Time: 5 minutes
Servings: 04

Ingredients :
- Coconut water, Servings cup

- Avocado, ½ hass

- Raw cacao, 2 teaspoons

- Vanilla, 1 teaspoon

- Dates, three (3)

- Sea salt, one (1) teaspoon

- Dark chocolate shavings

Directions:
1. Blend all Ingredients.

2. Blast until it becomes thick and smooth, as you wish.

3. Put in a fridge and allow it to get firm.

Nutrition:
Calories: 181.8

Fat: 151 g

Protein: 12 g

Chia Vanilla Coconut Pudding

Preparation Time: 5 minutes
Cooking Time: 5 minutes
Servings: 2

Ingredients :
• Coconut oil, 2 tablespoons

• Raw cashew, ½ cup

• Coconut water, ½ cup

• Cinnamon, 1 teaspoon

• Dates (pitted), 3

• Vanilla, 2 teaspoons

• Coconut flakes (unsweetened), 1 teaspoon

• Salt (Himalayan or Celtic Grey)

• Chia seeds, 6 tablespoons

• Cinnamon or pomegranate seeds for garnish (optional)

Directions:
1. Get a blender, add all the Ingredients (minus the pomegranate and chia seeds), and blend for about forty to sixty seconds.

2. Reduce the blender speed to the lowest and add the chia seeds.

3. Pour the content into an airtight container and put in a refrigerator for 25 minutes.

4. To serve, you can garnish with the cinnamon powder of pomegranate seeds.

Nutrition:
Calories: 201

Fat: 10 g

Sodium: 32.8 mg

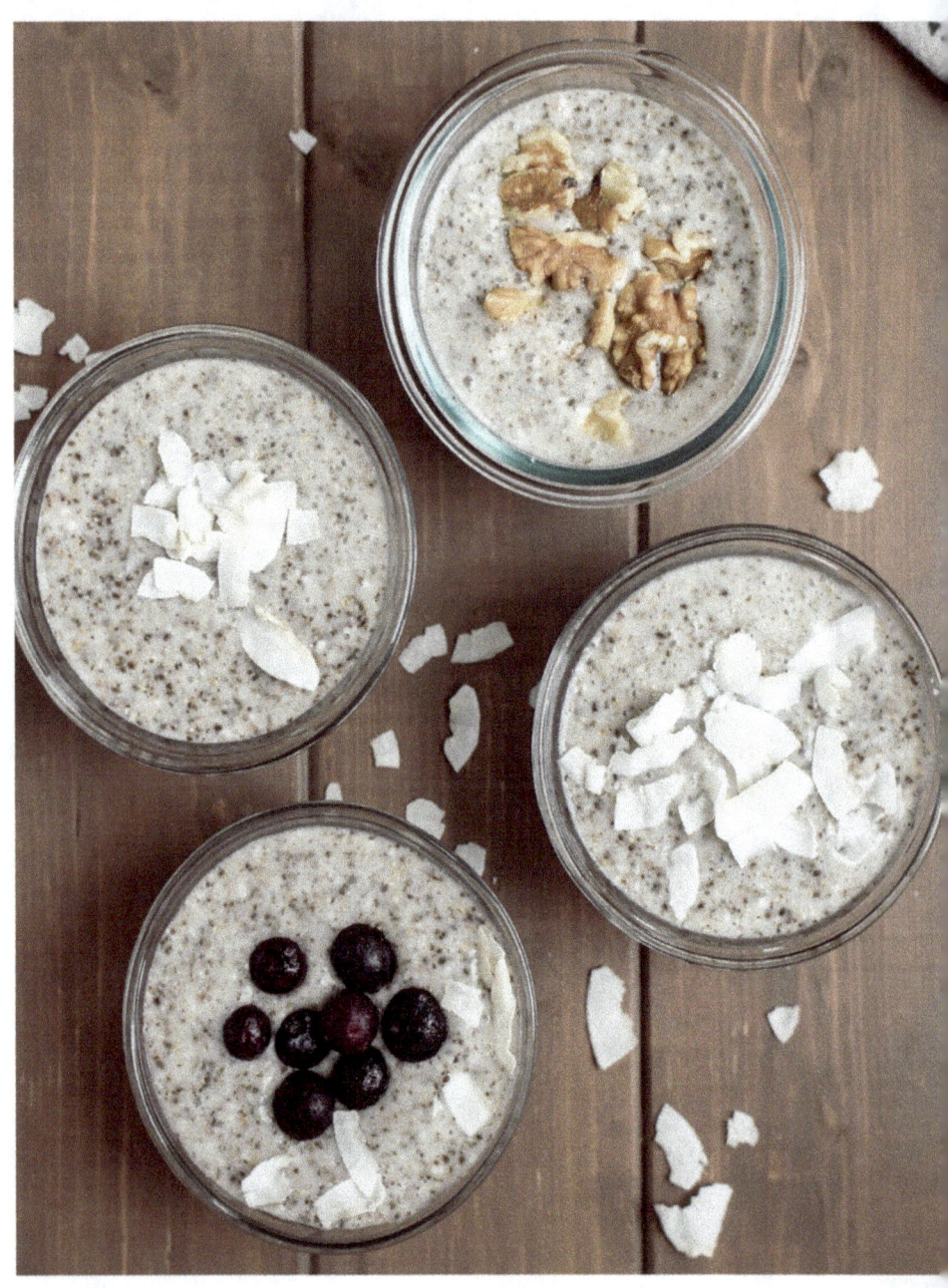

Sweet Tahini Dip With Ginger Cinnamon Fruit

Preparation Time: 10 minutes
Cooking Time: 5 minutes
Servings: 2

Ingredients :
- Cinnamon, one (1) teaspoon

- Green apple, one (1)

- Pear, one (1)

- Fresh ginger, two (2) – three (3)

- Celtic sea salt, one (1) teaspoon

- Ingredient for sweet Tahini

- Almond butter (raw), three (3) teaspoons

- Tahini (one big scoop), three (3) teaspoons

- Coconut oil, two (2) teaspoons

- Cayenne (optional), ¼ teaspoons

- Wheat-free tamari, two (2) teaspoons

- Liquid coconut nectar, one (1) teaspoon

Directions:
1. Get a clean mixing bowl.

2. Grate the ginger, add cinnamon, sea salt and mix together in the bowl.

3. Dice apple and pear into little cubes, turn into the bowl and mix.

4. Get a mixing bowl and mix all the Ingredients.

5. Then add the Sprinkle the Sweet Tahini Dip all over the Ginger Cinnamon Fruit.

6. Serve.

Nutrition:
Calories: 109

Fat: 10.8 g

Sodium: 258 mg

Coconut Butter And Chopped Berries With Mint

Preparation Time: 5 minutes
Cooking Time: 5 minutes
Servings: 04

Ingredients :
• Chopped mint, one (1) tablespoon

• Coconut butter (melted), two (2) tablespoons

• Mixed berries (strawberries, blueberries, and raspberries)

Directions:
1. Get a small bowl and add the berries.

2. Drizzle the melted coconut butter and sprinkle the mint.

3. Serve.

Nutrition:
Calories: 159

Fat: 12 g

Carbohydrates: 18 g

Alkaline Raw Pumpkin Pie

Preparation Time: 5 minutes
Cooking Time: 5 minutes
Servings: 04

Ingredients :
Ingredients for Pie Crust

- Cinnamon, one (1) teaspoon

- Dates/Turkish apricots, one (1) cup

- Raw almonds, one (1) cup

- Coconut flakes (unsweetened), one (1) cup

Ingredients for Pie Filling

- Dates, six (6)

- Cinnamon, ½ teaspoon

- Nutmeg, ½ teaspoon

- Pecans (soaked overnight), one (1) cup

- Organic pumpkin Blends (12 oz.), 1 ¼ cup

- Nutmeg, ½ teaspoon

- Sea salt (Himalayan or Celtic Sea Salt), ¼ teaspoon

- Vanilla, 1 teaspoon

- Gluten-free tamari

Directions:
Directions for pie crust

1. Get a food processor and blend all the pie crust Ingredients at the same time.

2. Make sure the mixture turns oily and sticky before you stop mixing.

3. Put the mixture in a pie pan and mold against the sides and floor, to make it stick properly.

Directions for the pie filling

1. Mix Ingredients together in a blender.

2. Add the mixture to fill in the pie crust.

3. Pour some cinnamon on top.

4. Then refrigerate till it's cold.

5. Then mold.

Nutrition:
Calories 135

Calories from Fat 41.4

Total Fat 4.6 g

Cholesterol 11.3 mg

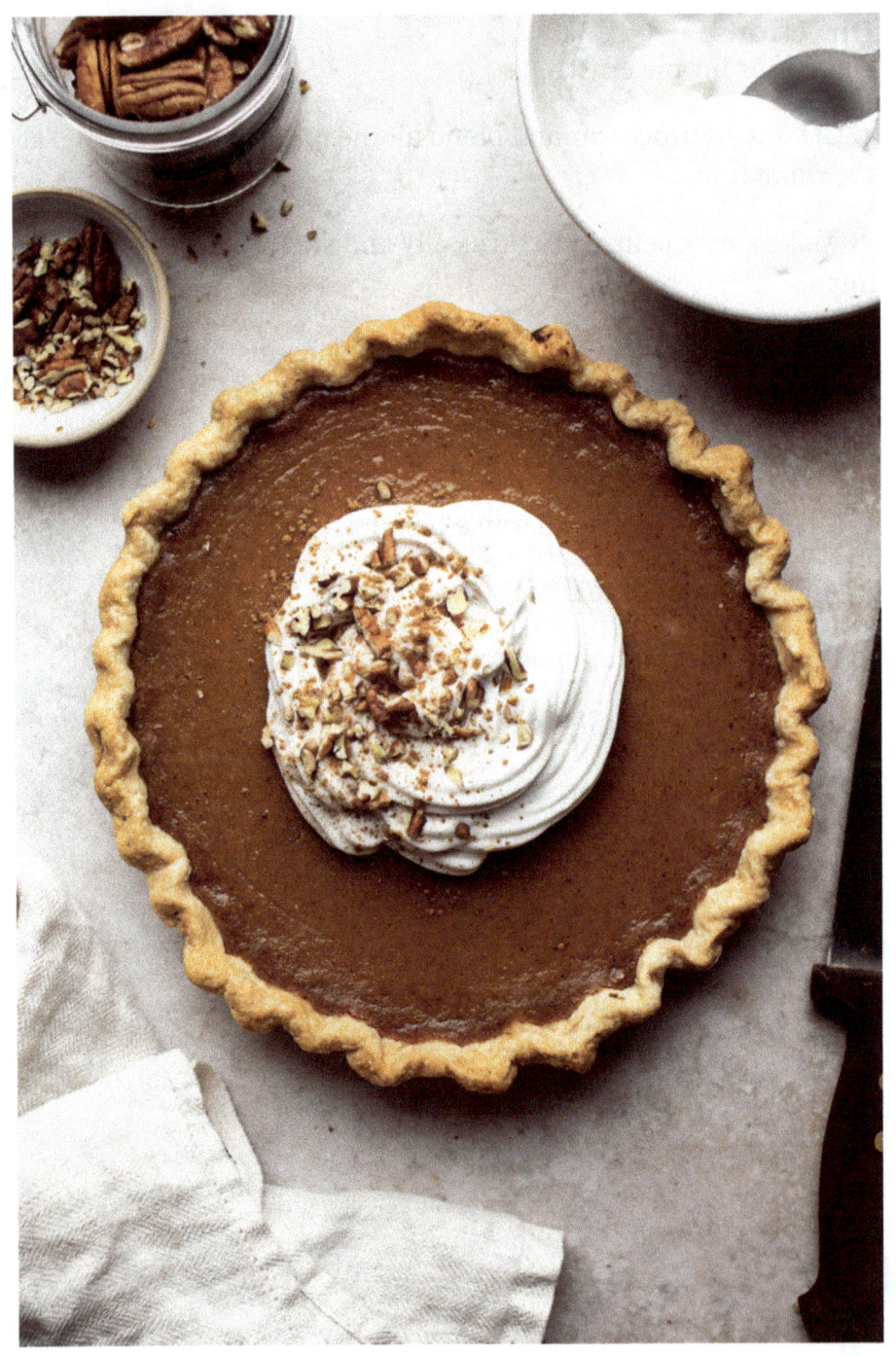

Strawberry Sorbet

Preparation Time: 5 minutes
Cooking Time: 40 minutes
Servings: 4

Ingredients :
- 2 cups of Strawberries*

- 1 1/2 teaspoons of Spelt Flour

- 1/2 cup of Date Sugar

- 2 cups of Spring Water

Directions:
- Add Date Sugar, Spring Water, and Spelt Flour to a medium pot and boil on low heat for about ten minutes. Mixture should thicken, like syrup.

- Remove the pot from the heat and allow it to cool.

- After cooling, add Blend Strawberry and mix gently.

- Put mixture in a container and freeze.

- Cut it into pieces, put the sorbet into a processor and blend until smooth.

- Put everything back in the container and leave in the refrigerator for at least 35 minutes.

- Serve and enjoy your Strawberry Sorbet!

Nutrition:
Calories: 198

Carbohydrates: 28 g

Blueberry Cupcakes

Preparation Time: 5 minutes
Cooking Time: 10 minutes
Servings: 3

Ingredients :
- 1/2 cup of Blueberries

- 3/4 cup of Teff Flour

- 3/4 cup of Spelt Flour

- 1/3 cup of Agave Syrup

- 1/2 teaspoon of Pure Sea Salt

- 1 cup of Coconut Milk

- 1/4 cup of Sea Moss Gel (optional, check information)

- Grape Seed Oil

Directions:
1. Preheat your oven to 365 degrees Fahrenheit.

2. Grease or line 6 standard muffin cups.

3. Add Teff, Spelt flour, Pure Sea Salt, Coconut Milk, Sea Moss Gel, and Agave Syrup to a large bowl. Mix them together.

4. Add Blueberries to the mixture and mix well.

5. Divide muffin batter among the 6 muffin cups.

6. Bake for 30 minutes until golden brown.

7. Serve and enjoy your Blueberry Muffins!

Nutrition:
Calories: 65

Fat: 0.7 g

Carbohydrates: 12 g

Protein: 1.4 g

Fiber: 5 g

Banana Strawberry Ice Cream

Preparation Time: 5 minutes
Cooking Time: 0 minutes
Servings: 5

Ingredients :
- 1 cup of Strawberry*

- 5 quartered Baby Bananas*

- 1/2 Avocado, chopped

- 1 tablespoon of Agave Syrup

- 1/4 cup of Homemade Walnut Milk

Directions:
1. Mix **Ingredients** into the blender and blend them well.

2. Taste. If it is too thick, add extra Milk or Agave Syrup if you want it sweeter.

3. Put in a container with a lid and allow to freeze for at least 35 minutes.

4. Serve it and enjoy your Banana Strawberry Ice Cream!

Nutrition:
Calories: 200

Fat: 0.5 g

Carbohydrates: 44 g

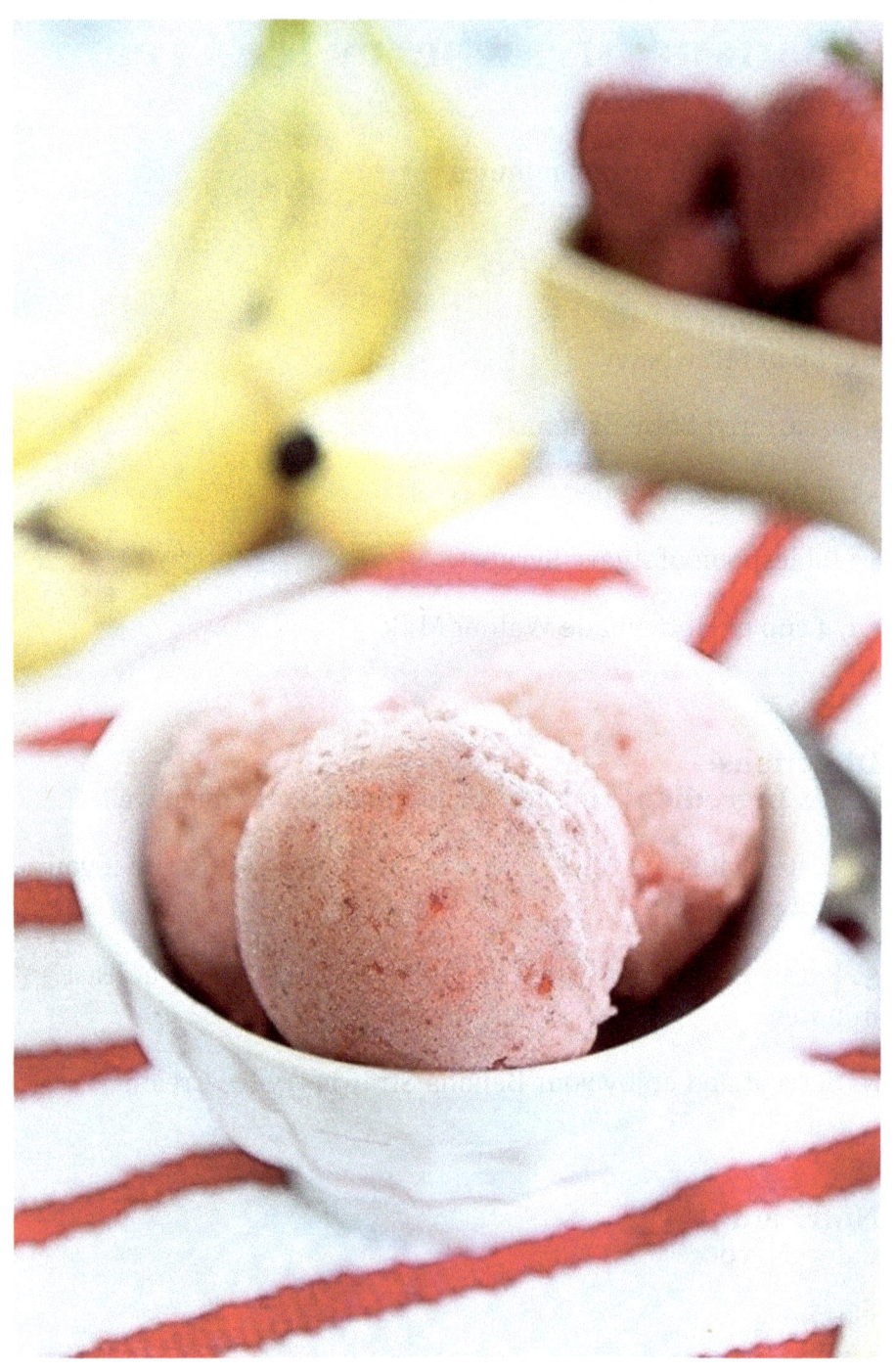

Homemade Whipped Cream

Preparation Time: 5 minutes
Cooking Time: 10 Minutes
Servings: 1 Cup

Ingredients :
- 1 cup of Aquafaba

- 1/4 cup of Agave Syrup

Directions:
1. Add Agave Syrup and Aquafaba into a bowl.

2. Mix at high speed around 5 minutes with a stand mixer or 10 to 15 minutes with a hand mixer.

3. Serve and enjoy your Homemade Whipped Cream!

Nutrition:
Calories: 21

Fat: 0g

Sodium: 0.3g

Carbohydrates: 5.3g

Fiber: 0g

Sugars: 4.7g

Protein: 0g

"Chocolate" Pudding

Preparation Time: 5 minutes
Cooking Time: 20 Minutes
Servings: 4

Ingredients :
- 1 to 2 cups of Black Sapote

- 1/4 cup of Agave Syrup

- 1/2 cup of soaked Brazil Nuts

- 1 tablespoon of Hemp Seeds

- 1/2 cup of Spring Water

Directions:

1. Cut 1 to 2 cups of Black Sapote in half.

2. Remove all seeds. You should have 1 full cup of de-seeded fruit.

3. Mix all Ingredients into a blender and blend until smooth.

4. Serve and enjoy your "Chocolate" Pudding!

Nutrition:
Calories: 134

Fat: 0.5 g

Carbohydrates: 15 g

Protein: 2.5 g

Fiber: 10 g

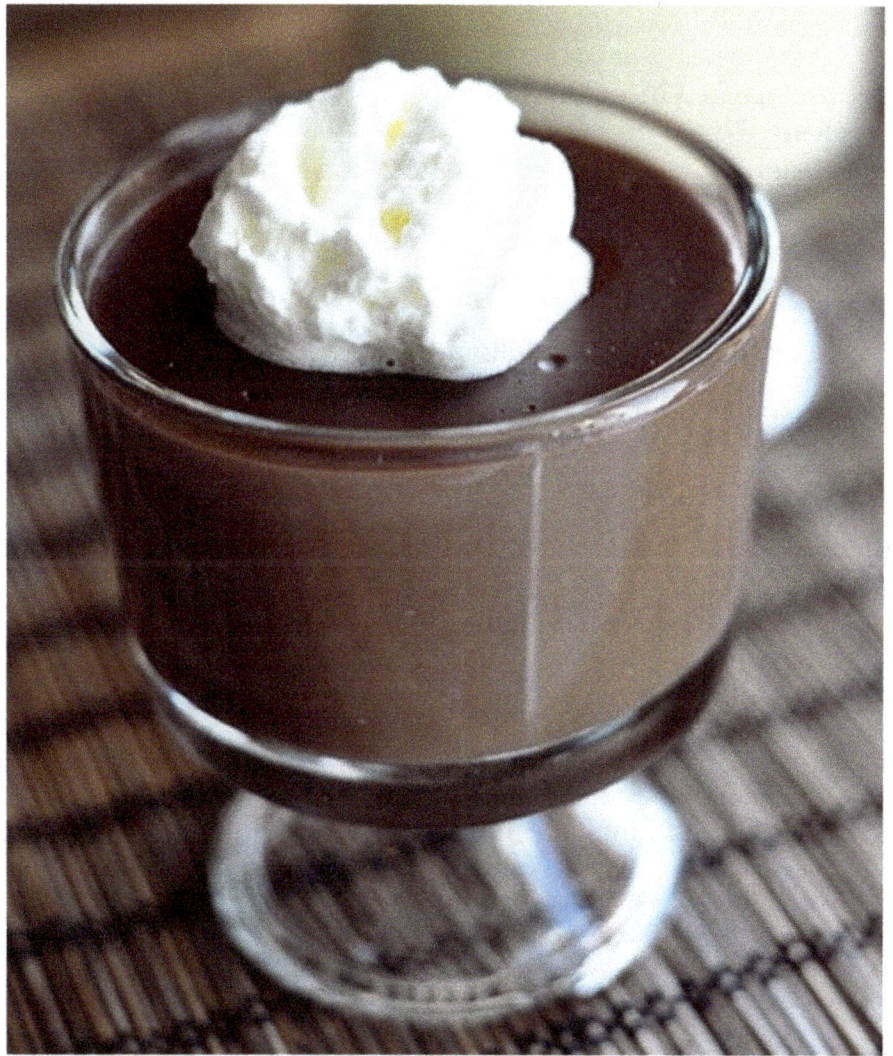

Banana Nut Muffins

Preparation Time: 5 minutes
Cooking Time: 30 minutes
Servings: 6

Ingredients
Dry Ingredients:

- 1 1/2 cups of Spell or Teff Flour

- 1/2 teaspoon of Pure Sea Salt

- 3/4 cup of Date Syrup

Wet Ingredients:

- 2 medium Blendd Burro Bananas

- ¼ cup of Grape Seed Oil

- ¾ cup of Homemade Walnut Milk (see recipe)*

- 1 tablespoon of Key Lime Juice

Filling Ingredients:

- ½ cup of chopped Walnuts (plus extra for decorating)

- 1 chopped Burro Banana

Directions:
1. Preheat your oven to 400 degrees Fahrenheit.

2. Take a muffin tray and grease 12 cups or line with cupcake liners.

3. Put all dry Ingredients in a large bowl and mix them thoroughly.

4. Add all wet Ingredients to a separate, smaller bowl and mix well with Blendd Bananas.

5. Mix Ingredients from the two bowls in one large container. Be careful not to over mix.

6. Add the filling Ingredients and fold in gently.

7. Pour muffin batter into the 12 prepared muffin cups and garnish with a couple Walnuts.

8. Bake it for 22 to 26 minutes until golden brown.

9. Allow to cool for 10 minutes.

10. Serve and enjoy your Banana Nut Muffins!

Nutrition:
Calories: 150

Fat: 10 g

Carbohydrates: 30 g

Protein: 2.4 g

Fiber: 2 g

Blackberry Jam

Preparation Time: 5 minutes
Cooking Time: 30 Minutes
Servings: 1 Cup

Ingredients :
• 3/4 cup of Blackberries

• 1 tablespoon of Key Lime Juice

• 3 tablespoons of Agave Syrup

• ¼ cup of Sea Moss Gel + extra 2 tablespoons (check information)

Directions:
1. Put rinsed Blackberries into a medium pot and cook on medium heat.

2. Stir Blackberries until liquid appears.

3. Once berries soften, use your immersion blender to chop up any large pieces. If you don't have a blender put the mixture in a food processor, mix it well, then return to the pot.

4. Add Sea Moss Gel, Key Lime Juice and Agave Syrup to the blended mixture. Boil on medium heat and stir well until it becomes thick.

5. Remove from the heat and leave it to cool for 10 minutes.

6. Serve it with bread pieces or the Flatbread (see recipe).

7. Enjoy your Blackberry Jam!

Nutrition:
Calories: 43

Fat: 0.5 g

Carbohydrates: 13 g

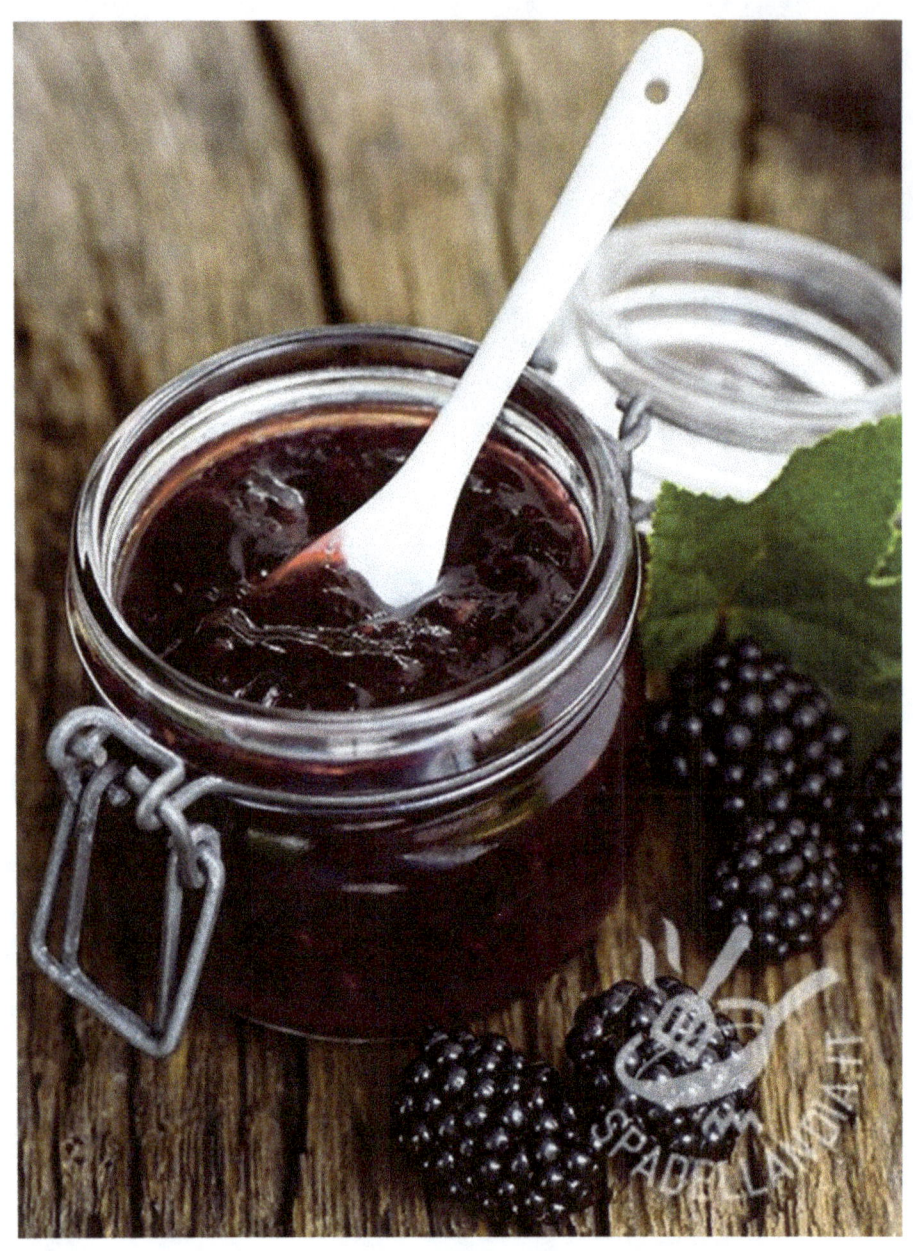

Blackberry Bars

Preparation Time: 5 minutes
Cooking Time: 20 Minutes
Servings: 4

Ingredients :
- 3 Burro Bananas or 4 Baby Bananas

- 1 cup of Spelt Flour

- 2 cups of Quinoa Flakes

- 1/4 cup of Agave Syrup

- 1/4 teaspoon of Pure Sea Salt

- 1/2 cup of Grape Seed Oil

- 1 cup of prepared Blackberry Jam

Directions:

1. Preheat your oven to 350 degrees Fahrenheit.

2. Remove skin of Bananas and mash with a fork in a large bowl.

3. Combine Agave Syrup and Grape Seed Oil with the Blend and mix well.

4. Add Spelt Flour and Quinoa Flakes. Knead the dough until it becomes sticky to your fingers.

5. Cover a 9x9-inch baking pan with parchment paper.

6. Take Servings of the dough and smooth it out over the parchment pan with your fingers.

7. Spread Blackberry Jam over the dough.

8. Crumble the remainder dough and sprinkle on the top.

9. Bake for 20 minutes.

10. Remove from the oven and let it cool for at 10 to 15 minutes.

11. Cut into small pieces.

12. Serve and enjoy your Blackberry Bars!

Nutrition:
Calories: 43

Fat: 0.5 g

Carbohydrates: 10 g

Protein: 1.4 g

Fiber: 5 g

Detox Berry Smoothie

Preparation Time: 15 minutes
Cooking Time: 0
Servings: 1

Ingredients :
- Spring water

- 1/4 avocado, pitted

- One medium burro banana

- One Seville orange

- Two cups of fresh lettuce

- One tablespoon of hemp seeds

- One cup of berries (blueberries or an aggregate of blueberries, strawberries, and raspberries)

Directions:
1. Add the spring water to your blender.

2. Put the fruits and vegies right inside the blender.

3. Blend all Ingredients till smooth.

Nutrition:
Calories: 202.4

Fat: 4.5g

Carbohydrates: 32.9g

Protein: 13.3g

Tabbouleh- Arabian Salad

Preparation Time: 5 minutes
Cooking Time: 10 minutes
Servings: 6

Ingredients :

- ¼ cup chopped fresh mint

- 1 **Servings:** cups boiling water

- 1 cucumber, peeled, seeded and chopped

- 1 cup bulgur

- 1 cup chopped fresh parsley

- 1 cup chopped green onions

- 1 tsp. salt

- 1/3 cup lemon juice

- 1/3 cup olive oil

- 3 tomatoes, chopped

- Ground black pepper to taste

Directions:

1. In a large bowl, mix together boiling water and bulgur. Let soak and set aside for an while covered.

2. After 10 minutes, toss in cucumber, tomatoes, mint, parsley, onions, lemon juice and oil. Then season with black pepper and salt to taste. Toss well and refrigerate for another 20 minutes while covered before serving.

Nutrition:
Calories: 185.5g

fat: 13.1g

Protein: 4.1g

Carbs: 12.8g

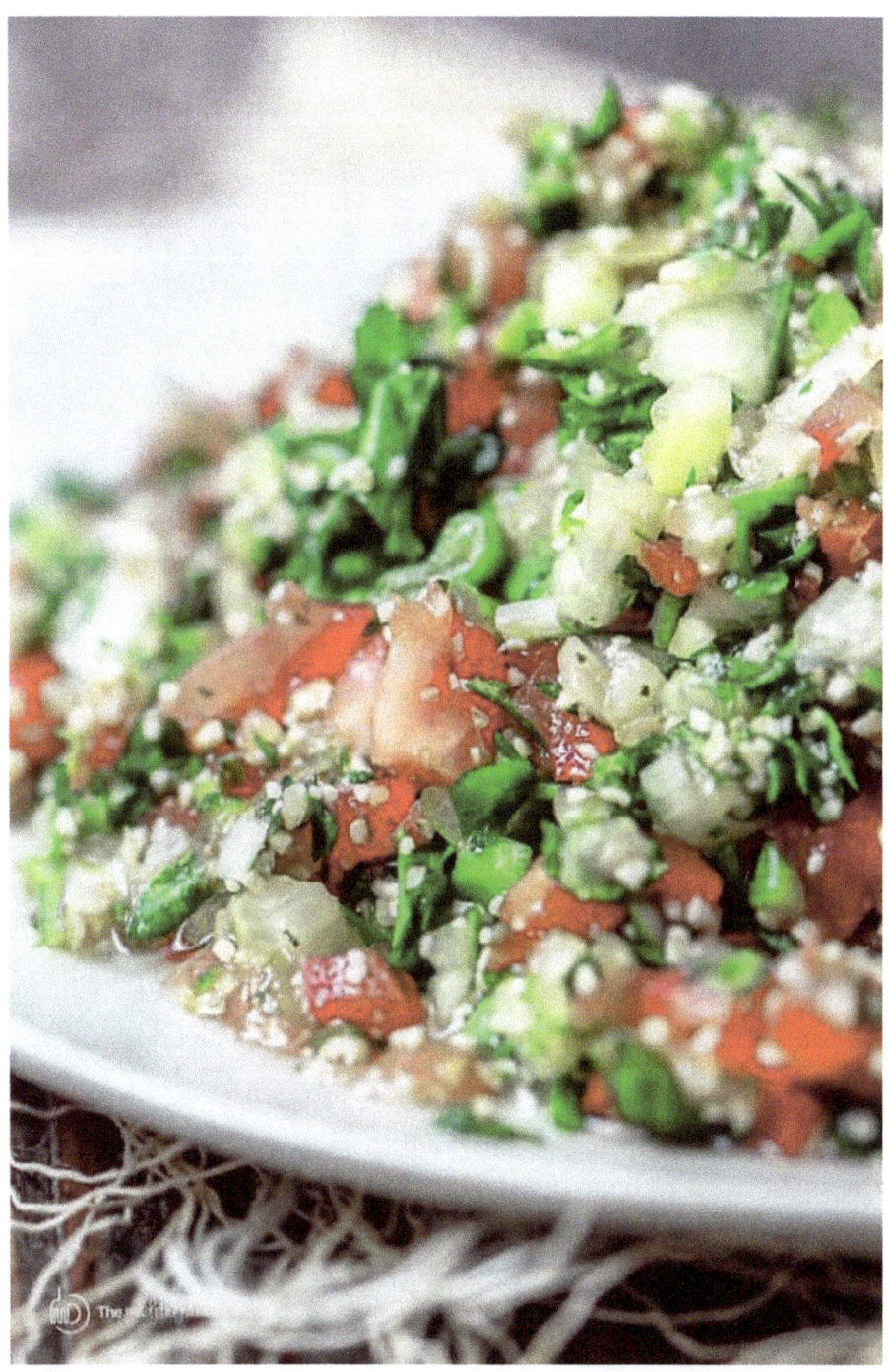

Aromatic Toasted Pumpkin Seeds

Preparation Time: 5 minutes
Cooking Time: 40 minutes
Servings: 4

Ingredients :
- 1 cup pumpkin seeds

- 1 teaspoon cinnamon

- 2 packets stevia

- 1 tablespoon canola oil

- ¼ teaspoon sea salt

Directions:
1. Prep the oven to 300°F (150°C).

2. Combine the pumpkin seeds with cinnamon, stevia, canola oil, and salt in a bowl. Stir to mix well.

3. Pour the seeds in the single layer on a baking sheet, then arrange the sheet in the preheated oven.

4. Bake for 40 minutes or until well toasted and fragrant. Shake the sheet twice to bake the seeds evenly.

5. Serve immediately.

Nutrition:
202 calories

5.1g carbohydrates

2.3g fiber

Bacon-Wrapped Shrimps

Preparation Time: 10 minutes
Cooking Time: 6 minutes
Servings: 10

Ingredient:

- 20 shrimps, peeled and deveined

- 7 slices bacon

- 4 leaves romaine lettuce

Directions:
1. Set the oven to 205°C.

2. Wrap each shrimp with each bacon strip, then arrange the wrapped shrimps in a single layer on a baking sheet, seam side down.

3. Broil for 6 minutes. Flip the shrimps halfway through the cooking time.

4. Take out from the oven and serve on lettuce leaves.

Nutrition:
70 calories

4.5g fat

7g protein

Cheesy Broccoli Bites

Preparation Time: 10 minutes
Cooking Time: 25 minutes
Servings: 6

Ingredient:

- 2 tablespoons olive oil

- 2 heads broccoli, trimmed

- 1 egg

- 1/3 cup reduced-fat shredded Cheddar cheese

- 1 egg white

- ½ cup onion, chopped

- 1/3 cup bread crumbs

- ¼ teaspoon salt

- ¼ teaspoon black pepper

Directions:
1. Ready the oven at 400°F (205°C). Coat a large baking sheet with olive oil.

2. Arrange a colander in a saucepan, then place the broccoli in the colander. Pour the water into the saucepan to cover the bottom. Boil, then reduce the heat to low. Close and simmer for 6 minutes. Allow cooling for 10 minutes.

3. Blend broccoli and remaining Ingredients in a food processor. Let sit for 10 minutes.

4. Make the bites: Drop 1 tablespoon of the mixture on the baking sheet. Repeat with the remaining mixture.

5. Bake in the preheated oven for 25 minutes. Flip the bites halfway through the cooking time.

6. Serve immediately.

Nutrition:
100 calories

13g carbohydrates

3g fiber

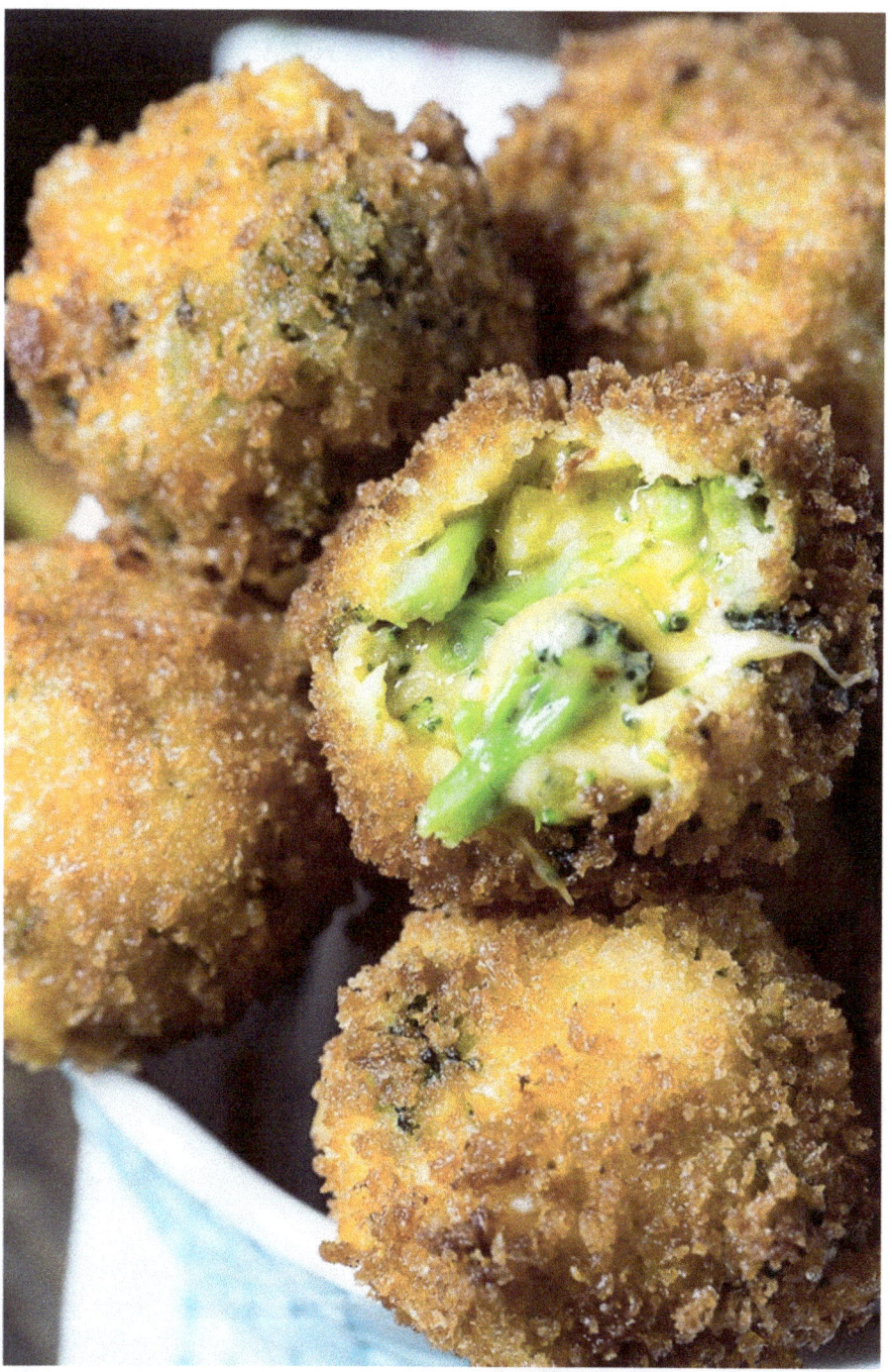

Easy Caprese Skewers

Preparation Time: 5 minutes
Cooking Time: 0 minute
Servings: 2

Ingredient:

- 12 cherry tomatoes

- 8 (1-inch) pieces Mozzarella cheese

- 12 basil leaves

- ¼ cup Italian Vinaigrette, for serving

Direction

1. Thread the tomatoes, cheese, and bay leave alternatively through the skewers.

2. Place the skewers on a huge plate and baste with the Italian Vinaigrette. Serve immediately.

Nutrition:
230 calories

8.5g carbohydrates

1.9g fiber

Grilled Tofu With Sesame Seeds

Preparation Time: 40 minutes
Cooking Time: 20 minutes
Servings: 6

Ingredient:

- 1½ tablespoons brown rice vinegar

- 1 scallion

- 1 tablespoon ginger root

- 1 tablespoon no-sugar-added applesauce

- 2 tablespoons naturally brewed soy sauce

- ¼ teaspoon dried red pepper flakes

- 2 teaspoons sesame oil, toasted

- 1 (14-ounce / 397-g) package extra-firm tofu

- 2 tablespoons fresh cilantro

- 1 teaspoon sesame seeds

Directions:
1. Combine the vinegar, scallion, ginger, applesauce, soy sauce, red pepper flakes, and sesame oil in a large bowl. Stir to mix well.

2. Dunk the tofu pieces in the bowl, then refrigerate to marinate for 30 minutes.

3. Preheat a grill pan over medium-high heat.

4. Place the tofu on the grill pan with tongs, reserve the marinade, then grill for 8 minutes or until the tofu is golden brown and have deep grilled marks on both sides. Flip the tofu halfway through the cooking time. You may need to work in batches to avoid overcrowding.

5. Transfer the tofu to a large plate and sprinkle with cilantro leaves and sesame seeds. Serve with the marinade alongside.

Nutrition:
90 calories

3g carbohydrates

1g fiber

Kale Chips

Preparation Time: 5 minutes
Cooking Time: 15 minutes
Servings: 1

Ingredients :
- ¼ teaspoon garlic powder

- Pinch cayenne to taste

- 1 tablespoon extra-virgin olive oil

- ½ teaspoon sea salt, or to taste

- 1 (8-ounce) bunch kale

Directions:
1. Prepare oven at 180°C. Line two baking sheets with parchment paper.

2. Toss the garlic powder, cayenne pepper, olive oil, and salt in a large bowl, then dunk the kale in the bowl.

3. Situate kale in a single layer on one of the baking sheets.

4. Arrange the sheet in the preheated oven and bake for 7 minutes. Remove the sheet from the oven and pour the kale into the single layer of the other baking sheet.

5. Move the sheet of kale back to the oven and bake for another 7 minutes.

6. Serve immediately.

Nutrition

136 calories

3g carbohydrates

1.1g fiber

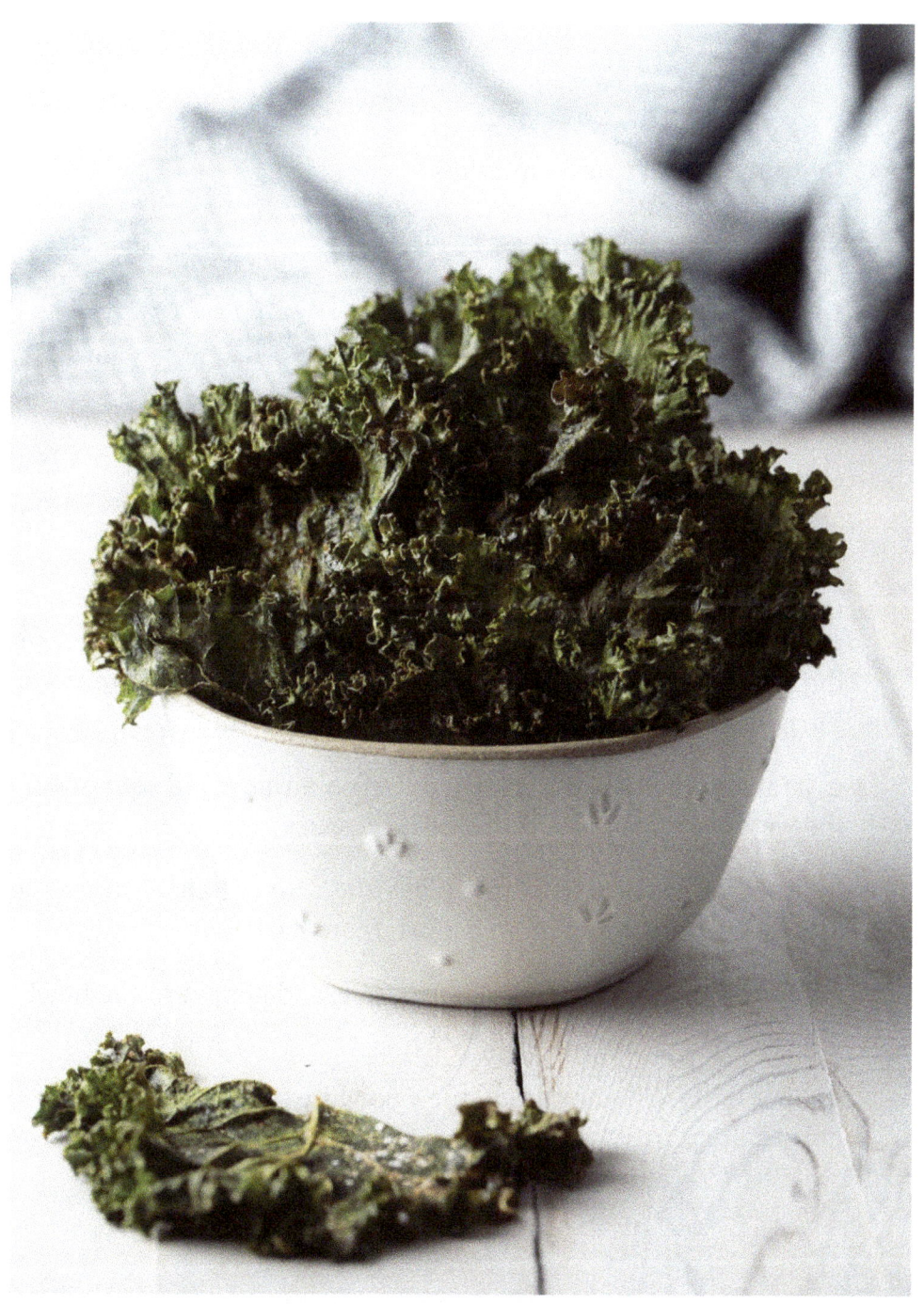

Simple Deviled Eggs

Preparation Time: 5 minutes
Cooking Time: 8 minutes
Servings: 12

Ingredients :
• 6 large eggs

• 1/8 teaspoon mustard powder

• 2 tablespoons light mayonnaise

Directions:
1. Sit the eggs in a saucepan, then pour in enough water to cover the egg. Bring to a boil, then boil the eggs for another 8 minutes. Turn off the heat and cover, then let sit for 15 minutes.

2. Transfer the boiled eggs to a pot of cold water and peel under the water.

3. Transfer the eggs to a large plate, then cut in half. Remove the egg yolks and place them in a bowl, then mash with a fork.

4. Add the mustard powder, mayo, salt, and pepper to the bowl of yolks, then stir to mix well.

5. Spoon the yolk mixture in the egg white on the plate. Serve immediately.

Nutrition:
45 calories

1g carbohydrates

0.9g fiber

Sautéed Collard Greens And Cabbage

Preparation Time: 10 minutes
Cooking Time: 10 minutes
Servings: 8

Ingredients :
- 2 tablespoons extra-virgin olive oil

- 1 collard greens bunch

- ½ small green cabbage

- 6 garlic cloves

- 1 tablespoon low-sodium soy sauce

Directions:
1. Cook olive oil in a large skillet over medium-high heat.

2. Sauté the collard greens in the oil for about 2 minutes, or until the greens start to wilt.

3. Toss in the cabbage and mix well. Set to medium-low, cover, and cook for 5 to 7 minutes, stirring occasionally, or until the greens are softened.

4. Fold in the garlic and soy sauce and stir to combine. Cook for about 30 seconds more until fragrant.

5. Remove from the heat to a plate and serve.

Nutrition:
73 calories

5.9g carbohydrates

2.9g fiber

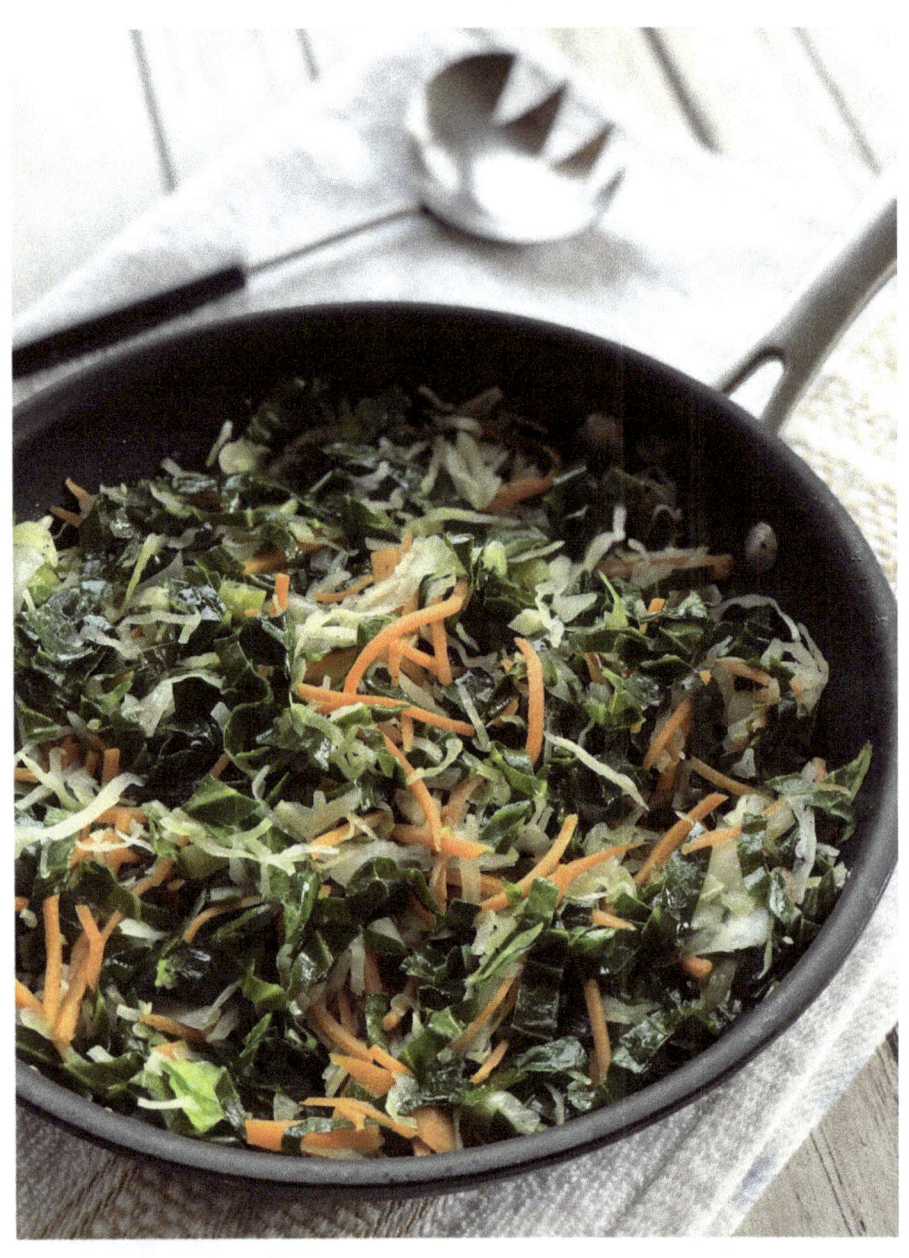

Roasted Delicata Squash With Thyme

Preparation Time: 10 minutes
Cooking Time: 20 minutes
Servings: 4

Ingredients :
- 1 (1½-pound) Delicata squash
- 1 tablespoon extra-virgin olive oil
- ½ teaspoon dried thyme
- ¼ teaspoon salt
- ¼ teaspoon freshly ground black pepper

Directions:
1. Prep the oven to 400°F (205°C). Ready baking sheet with parchment paper and set aside.

2. Add the squash strips, olive oil, thyme, salt, and pepper in a large bowl, and toss until the squash strips are fully coated.

3. Place the squash strips on the prepared baking sheet in a single layer. Roast for about 20 minutes, flipping the strips halfway through.

4. Remove from the oven and serve on plates.

Nutrition:
78 calories

11.8g carbohydrates

2.1g fiber

Roasted Asparagus And Red Peppers

Preparation Time: 5 minutes
Cooking Time: 15 minutes
Servings: 4

Ingredients :
- 1-pound (454 g) asparagus

- 2 red bell peppers, seeded

- 1 small onion

- 2 tablespoons Italian dressing

Directions:
1. Ready oven to (205ºC). Wrap baking sheet with parchment paper and set aside.

2. Combine the asparagus with the peppers, onion, dressing in a large bowl, and toss well.

3. Arrange the vegetables on the baking sheet and roast for about 15 minutes. Flip the vegetables with a spatula once during cooking.

4. Transfer to a large platter and serve.

Nutrition:
92 calories

10.7g carbohydrates

4g fiber

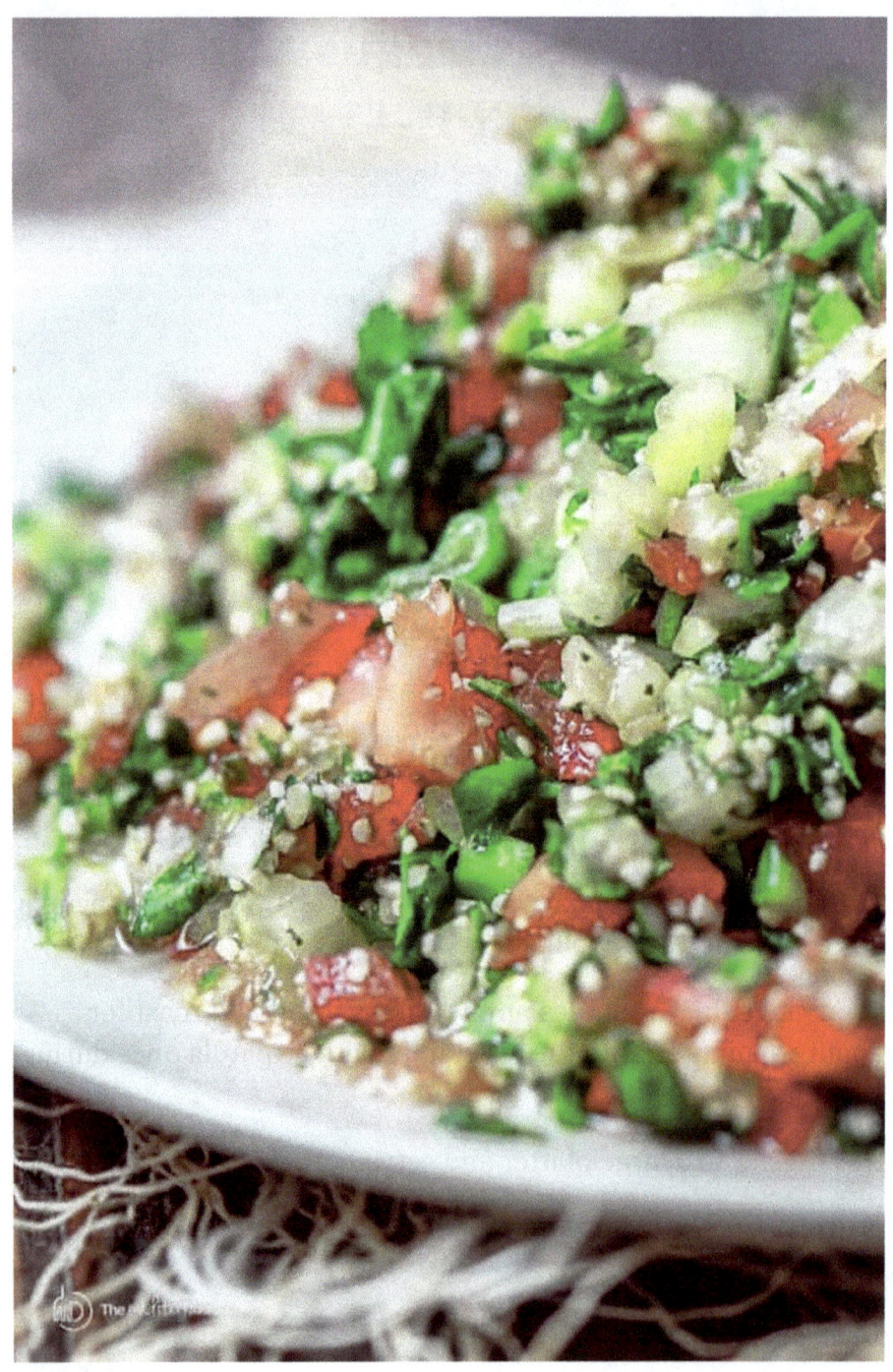

Tarragon Spring Peas

Preparation Time: 10 minutes
Cooking Time: 12 minutes
Servings: 6

Ingredients :
1 tablespoon unsalted butter

½ Vidalia onion

1 cup low-sodium vegetable broth

3 cups fresh shelled peas

1 tablespoon minced fresh tarragon

Directions:
1. Cook butter in a pan at medium heat.

2. Sauté the onion in the melted butter for about 3 minutes, stirring occasionally.

3. Pour in the vegetable broth and whisk well. Add the peas and tarragon to the skillet and stir to combine.

4. Reduce the heat to low, cover, cook for about 8 minutes more, or until the peas are tender.

5. Let the peas cool for 5 minutes and serve warm.

Nutrition:
82 calories

12g carbohydrates

3.8g fiber

Butter-Orange Yams

Preparation Time: 7 minutes
Cooking Time: 40 minutes
Servings: 8

Ingredients :
- 2 medium jewel yams

- 2 tablespoons unsalted butter

- Juice of 1 large orange

- 1½ teaspoons ground cinnamon

- ¼ teaspoon ground ginger

- ¾ teaspoon ground nutmeg

- 1/8 teaspoon ground cloves

Directions:
1. Set oven at 180°C.

2. Arrange the yam dices on a rimmed baking sheet in a single layer. Set aside.

3. Add the butter, orange juice, cinnamon, ginger, nutmeg, and garlic cloves to a medium saucepan over medium-low heat. Cook for 3 to 5 minutes, stirring continuously.

4. Spoon the sauce over the yams and toss to coat well.

5. Bake in the prepared oven for 40 minutes.

6. Let the yams cool for 8 minutes on the baking sheet before removing and serving.

Nutrition:
129 calories

24.7g carbohydrates

5g fiber

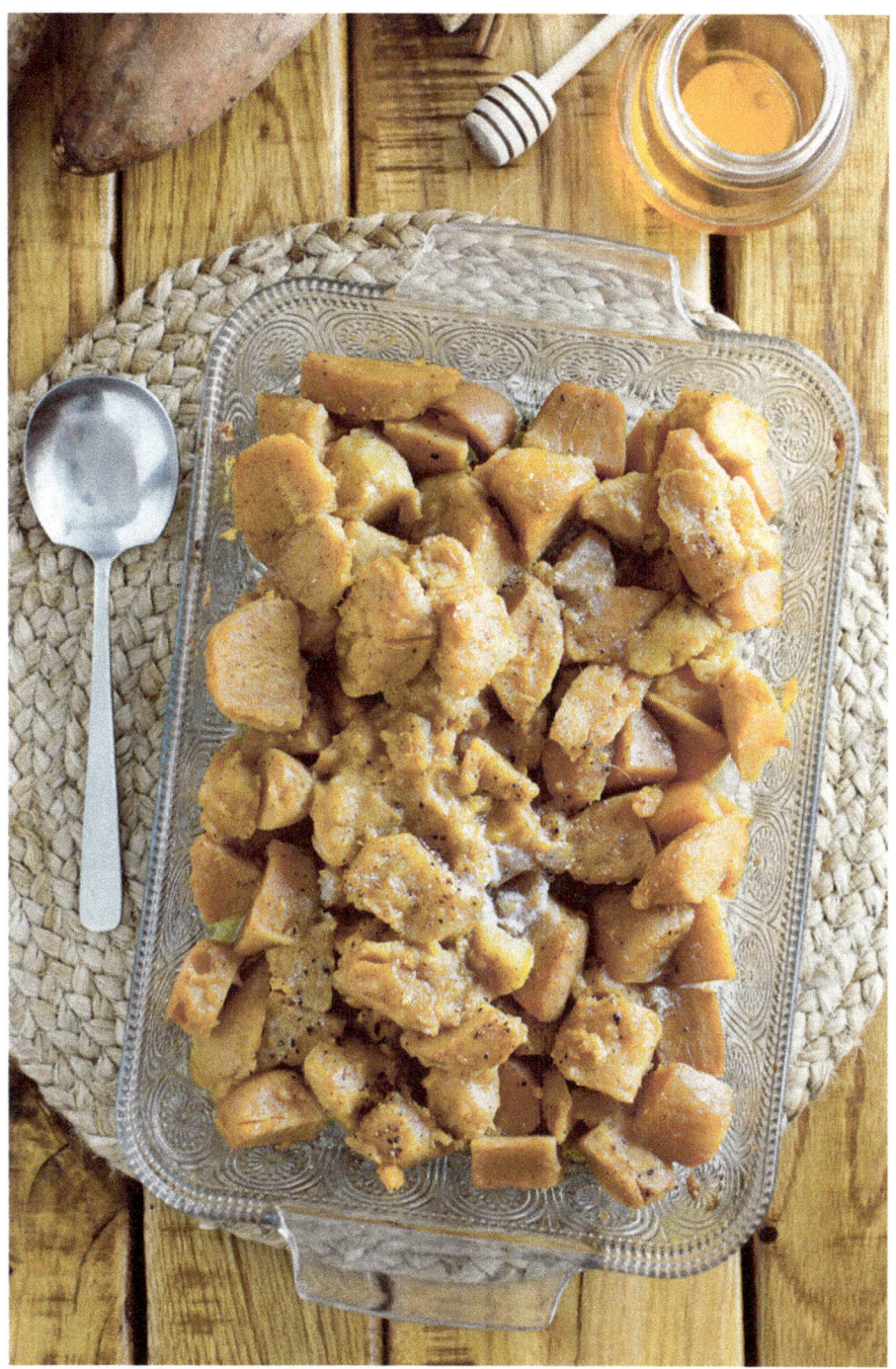

Roasted Tomato Brussels Sprouts

Preparation Time: 15 minutes
Cooking Time: 20 minutes
Servings: 4

Ingredients :
- 1-pound (454 g) Brussels sprouts

- 1 tablespoon extra-virgin olive oil

- ½ cup sun-dried tomatoes

- 2 tablespoons lemon juice

- 1 teaspoon lemon zest

Directions:
1. Set oven 205°C. Prep large baking sheet with aluminum foil.

2. Toss the Brussels sprouts in the olive oil in a large bowl until well coated. Sprinkle with salt and pepper.

3. Spread out the seasoned Brussels sprouts on the prepared baking sheet in a single layer.

4. Roast for 20 minutes, shake halfway through.

5. Remove from the oven then situate in a bowl. Whisk tomatoes, lemon juice, and lemon zest, to incorporate. Serve immediately.

Nutrition:
111 calories

13.7g carbohydrates

4.9g fiber

Simple Sautéed Greens

Preparation Time: 10 minutes
Cooking Time: 10 minutes
Servings: 4

Ingredients :
- 2 tablespoons extra-virgin olive oil

- 1 pound (454 g) Swiss chard

- 1-pound (454 g) kale

- ½ teaspoon ground cardamom

- 1 tablespoon lemon juice

Directions:
1. Heat up olive oil in a big skillet over medium-high heat.

2. Stir in Swiss chard, kale, cardamom, lemon juice to the skillet, and stir to combine. Cook for about 10 minutes, stirring continuously, or until the greens are wilted.

3. Sprinkle with the salt and pepper and stir well.

4. Serve the greens on a plate while warm.

Nutrition:
139 calories

15.8g carbohydrates

3.9g fiber

Garlicky Mushrooms

Preparation Time: 10 minutes
Cooking Time: 12 minutes
Servings: 4

Ingredients :
- 1 tablespoon butter

- 2 teaspoons extra-virgin olive oil

- 2 pounds button mushrooms

- 2 teaspoons minced fresh garlic

- 1 teaspoon chopped fresh thyme

Directions:
1. Warm up butter and olive oil in a huge skillet over medium-high heat.

2. Add the mushrooms and sauté for 10 minutes, stirring occasionally.

3. Stir in the garlic and thyme and cook for an additional 2 minutes.

4. Season and serve on a plate.

Nutrition:
96 calories

8.2g carbohydrates

1.7g fiber

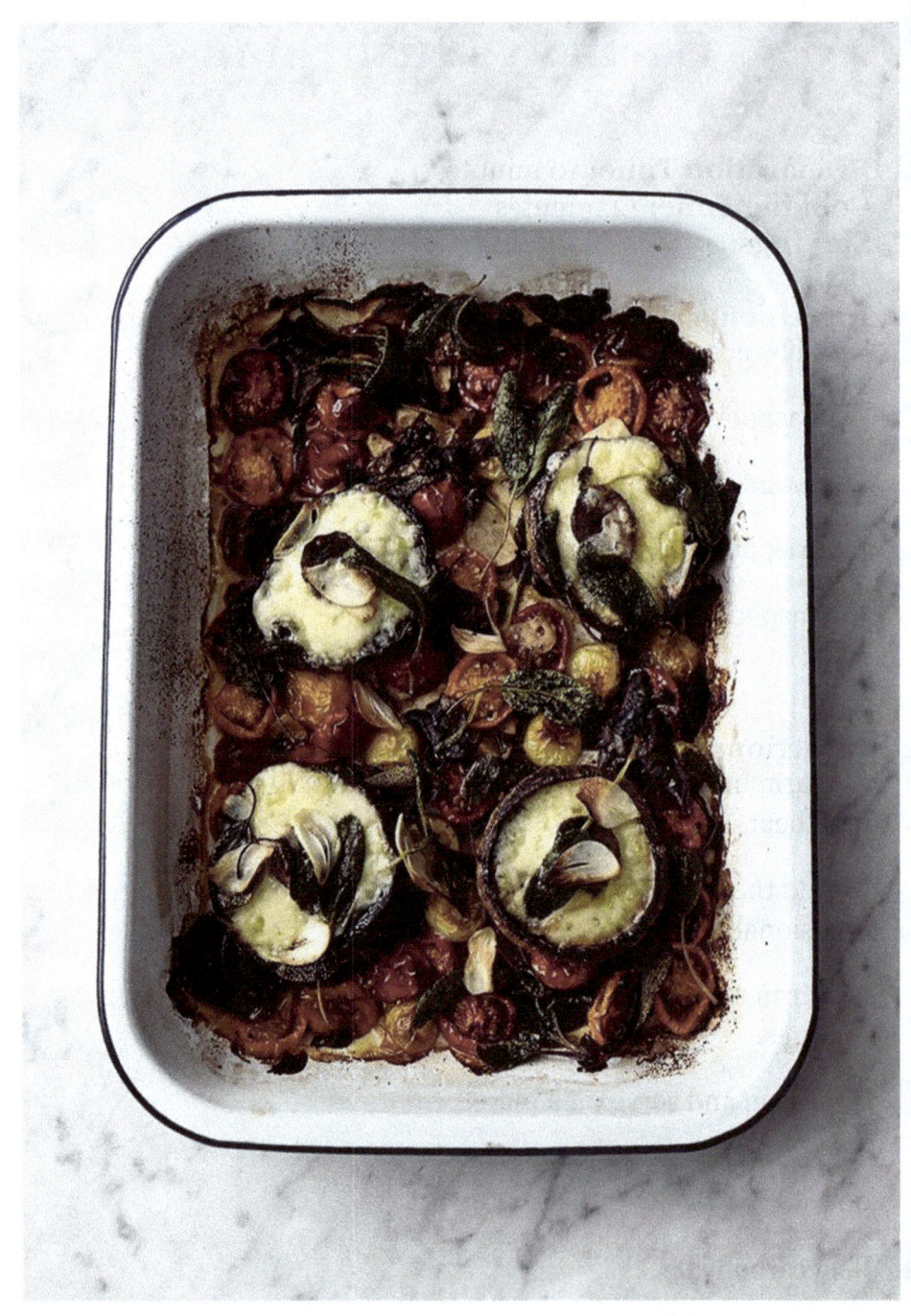

www.ingramcontent.com/pod-product-compliance
Lightning Source LLC
Chambersburg PA
CBHW070725030426
42336CB00013B/1916